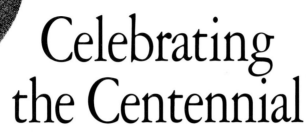

Celebrating
the Centennial
1892 - 1992

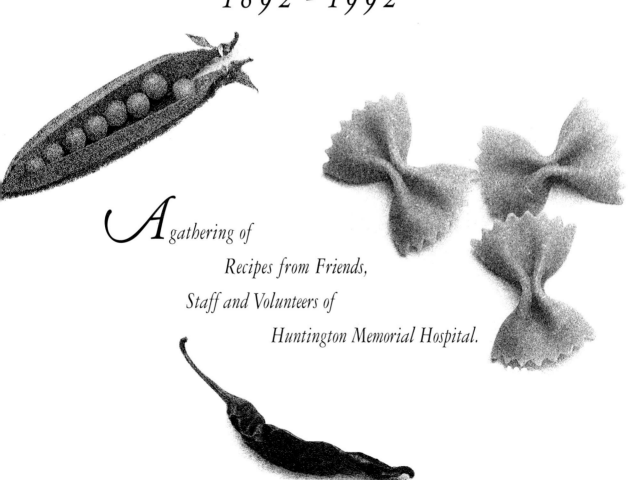

*A gathering of
Recipes from Friends,
Staff and Volunteers of
Huntington Memorial Hospital.*

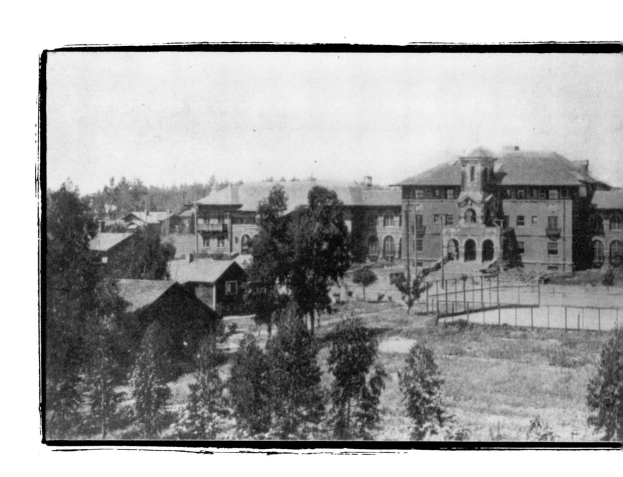

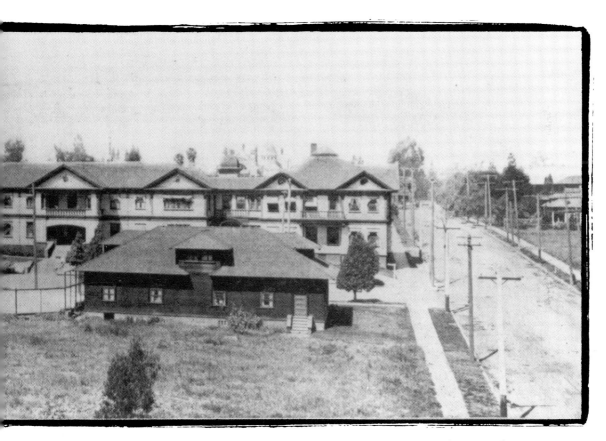

Pasadena Hospital, circa 1908 - 1909

The proceeds realized from the sale of "Celebrating the Centennial"
will be returned to Huntington Memorial Hospital,
specifically to improve and enhance the Courtyard-an open area for all to enjoy.

Additional copies of "Celebrating the Centennial"
may be obtained by writing: "Celebrating the Centennial"
                              Volunteer Services
                              Huntington Memorial Hospital
                              100 West California Boulevard
                              Pasadena, California 91105

Please enclose your return address with a check payable to
Huntington Memorial Hospital Cookbook in the amount of $22.50
per book plus, $3.00 postage and handling.
California residents add $1.85 sales tax per book.

First Printing, September 1991
Printed by: Green Street Press
              1070 East Green Street
              Pasadcna, California 91106

The caring spirit which was the driving force behind this commemorative Centennial Cookbook has been an inspiration to those of us who falter when tenacity, creativity, and constant dialogue are required to complete an assignment! For the three-and-a-half years of work which preceded the final printing, the cookbook committee diligently planned, tested recipes, and successfully raised money to fund this book. Boutiques and bake sales, raffles and holiday baskets were among the many fund-raising efforts which helped make this book a reality. We are deeply grateful to all of the committee for this wonderful contribution to our centennial year. We congratulate them for their constancy, diligence and love which provided us with this celebratory book. I am confident that the following pages will communicate the commitment and joy that are the embodiment of the Centennial Cookbook Committee.

Elsie Sadler

Elsie Sadler
Director of Development and Public Relations

It is with great pleasure that we dedicate "Celebrating the Centennial" Cookbook to the employees, volunteers and friends of Huntington Memorial Hospital, whose participation and contribution of talent and time made this publication a reality.

Co-Chairman: Charmaine Carter and Jean-Anne Hawley

Treasurer: Dorothy Hull

Secretary: Dorothy Marshall

Cookbook Steering Committee:

Cathy Andrews	Beverly Levin
Holly Bennett	Wyllis Leonhard
Judy Bolenbaugh	Elizabeth Little
Melia Bressler	Peggy Logan
Marty Crick	Bobbie Miller
Linda Cseak	Charlotte Packard
Carole DePaul	Mary Pavlinek
Loretta Dito	Diane Rinaldi
Dorothy Duer	Jewell Rosier
Sue Fender	Peggy Russell
Dottie Juett	Gay Sanborn
Virginia Khazoyan	Maureen Savage
Miriam Kipnis	Susan Seitz
Leah Kurihara	Maura Walsh

Huntington Memorial Hospital Advisors:

Dawn Dattola	Peg Kean
Priscilla Gamb	Elsie Sadler
Geri Hamane	Debra Weigand
Anne James	

Design: Art Center College of Design: Dean Sprague and Marcus Greinke
Cover Design: Lindon Gray Leader Corporate Design

Special thanks to Wyllis Leonhard for her generous donation.

Table of Contents

§ *Denotes recipes with nutritional information*

*I*n the early days of Pasadena, getting adequate medical care for serious illness meant a long, bumpy ride in a Southern Pacific baggage car to Los Angeles. So, in February 1892, a group of prominent citizens formed the Pasadena Hospital Association with the goal of providing a medical facility for Pasadena. In 1899, the first patient was admitted to temporary headquarters, and the non-profit organization supported itself with donations, membership dues and patient fees. In 1900, a committee was appointed to raise funds to build and endow a permanent hospital building. Two years later a 26-bed facility opened at the present site of Huntington Memorial Hospital. The hospital grew over the years, but by the late 1920's had fallen on hard times. In 1936, a $2,000,000 gift by the late Henry E. Huntington gave the hospital a new beginning and its current name: the Collis P. and Howard Huntington Memorial Hospital. From these beginnings, Huntington Memorial Hospital has become a non-profit, 606-bed facility dedicated to providing full-service, state-of-the-art medical care to the San Gabriel Valley communities. As we celebrate our centennial, we wish to acknowledge all who came before us for their foresight, support and dedication. For the next one hundred years, Huntington Memorial Hospital is committed to responding to the needs of the community and providing the best of care for life.

Allen W. Mathies, Jr., M.D.
President and Chief Executive Officer

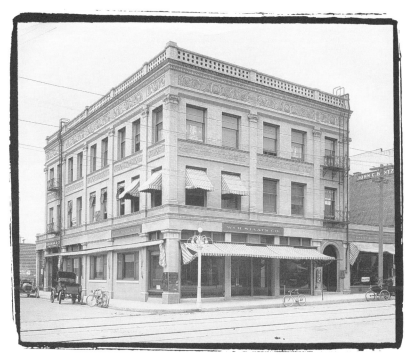

Site of hospital's first temporary facilities (1899 - 1902)

hors d'oeurves and beverages

Lemon Syrup

Take the juice of twelve lemons; grate the rind of six in it, let it stand over night; then take six pounds of white sugar and make a thick syrup. When it is quite cool, strain the juice into it, and squeeze as much oil from the grated rind as will suit the taste.

Put in bottles, securely corked, for future use. A tablespoonful in a goblet of water will make a delicious drink on a hot day.

The White House Cookbook © 1887

Artichoke Quiche

6 to 8 servings.

2 jars marinated artichoke hearts,
chopped
1 onion, chopped
5 eggs
½ cup bread crumbs
2 cups grated cheddar cheese
Italian seasoning of your choice

Drain marinade from artichokes into a small skillet. Cook onion in artichoke oil until limp. Add artichoke hearts and cook 5 minutes more. Mix remaining ingredients along with above mixture. Pour mixture into a greased 9″ x 9″ pan and bake in 350 degree oven for 30 minutes or until golden brown.

Chinese Fritters

36 fritters.

6 eggs
1 cup flour
1½ teaspoons baking powder
½ teaspoon salt
1 tablespoon soy sauce
½ teaspoon Worcestershire sauce
1 16 ounce can bean sprouts,
well drained and snipped with scissors
1 envelope onion soup mix
1 4 ounce can mushroom stems and
pieces, well drained
1 1.5 ounce can shrimp,
well drained and chopped
1 8 ounce can water chestnuts,
drained and chopped

Beat eggs slightly, and add other ingredients in order given. Drop by teaspoonfuls into ½″ hot vegetable oil that has been preheated to 375 degrees in an electric skillet or deep fryer. Fry for 2-3 minutes on each side. Drain on paper towels.

Popeye's Hot Spinach Dip

6 cups.

2 cups ricotta, part-skim ricotta or
light ricotta cheese
1 cup sour cream
1 10 ounce package frozen chopped
spinach, thawed and well-drained
¼ pound diced ham
¾ cup shredded parmesan cheese
½ cup chopped green onions
1 round loaf bread, unsliced

In food processor, blender or electric mixer, combine ricotta cheese and sour cream; process until smooth. Stir in spinach, ham, parmesan cheese and green onions. Cut 1″ slice off top of bread; reserve. Remove bread from inside loaf, retaining 1¾″ shell; cut bread from inside loaf into bite-size cubes.

Pour cheese mixture into bread shell; replace top, wrap in foil and place on baking sheet. Bake in 350 degree oven 1 hour 15 minutes or until heated through.

Arrange bread loaf and bread cubes on large serving platter.

Betsy's Hot Rounds

24 servings.

½ bunch green onions, chopped
½ cup parmesan cheese
5-6 drops tabasco
1 cup mayonnaise
Bread rounds, stale

Mix first 4 ingredients together. Spread on stale bread rounds. Place on cookie sheet. Heat oven to 350 degrees and bake for 10 minutes. Serve immediately.

Cocktails Fiesta

100 appetizers.

1 pound grated Tillamook cheese or mild cheddar
1 can tomato sauce
2 cans chopped ripe olives
½ cup vegetable oil
Salt to taste
3 hard boiled eggs, chopped
6 green onions, chopped
2 cloves garlic, minced
1 4 ounce can diced green chiles
Crackers

Mix all ingredients together, except crackers, and freeze. To serve, place ½ teaspoon of cheese mixture on each cracker and put in 350 degree oven for 10 minutes. Serve immediately.

Bread Spread

4 dozen.

4 ounces diced green chiles
¼ pound butter, softened to room temperature
1 cup mayonnaise
½ pound Monterey Jack cheese, grated
2 loaves French bread, small diameter
Cilantro or parsley, chopped

In medium bowl, mix chiles, butter, mayonnaise and cheese until well blended. Slice French bread into thin slices and spread with cheese mixture, completely covering bread. Place slices on ungreased cookie sheet. Broil about 5 minutes until spread is bubbly. Garnish with parsley or cilantro.

Cheese Bread Rolls

20 servings.

1 large loaf sliced white sandwich bread
1 pound sharp cheese, grated
1 tablespoon Worcestershire sauce
Minced dry onion
8 tablespoons margarine
½ cup mayonnaise
Minced parsley

Trim off crust; roll each slice flat with rolling pin. Combine remaining ingredients. Spread portion of mixture on bread slice and roll. Place each roll seam down on cookie sheet. Toast in 400 degree oven for 12 minutes. Can be frozen and cooked at last minute.

Cream Cheese Crab Spread

20 servings.

1 8 ounce package cream cheese
4 green onions, chopped
1 teaspoon lemon juice
1 7.5 ounce can drained crab
½ cup catsup
1 tablespoon horseradish

Combine cream cheese, onions, lemon juice and crab. Mix well and let set in refrigerator to blend flavors, all day if possible. Mix catsup and horseradish together. Serve spreads in separate bowls or layer catsup mixture over crab spread. Serve with crackers.

Crab Cheese Appetizer

12 servings.

1 round unsliced loaf sourdough
bread uncut
1 pound velveeta cheese
1 cup sour cream
2 teaspoons Worcestershire sauce
1 cup mayonnaise
1 teaspoon cayenne pepper
½ pound crab meat

Cut 'lid' from top of sourdough loaf. Hollow out bread from remaining loaf to form a cavity. Cut hollowed-out bread into dipping-sized pieces. Toast them in oven.

Melt the velveeta cheese. Mix together the sour cream, Worcestershire sauce, mayonnaise, cayenne pepper and crab meat. Add to the melted cheese.

Pour into hollow cavity of bread loaf and cover with bread lid. Bake in 350 degree oven for 1 hour.

E-Z Tiny Meatballs

10 servings.

1 12 ounce bottle chili sauce
1 16 ounce can whole cranberries
1 chopped onion or
½ cup dehydrated onion
1½ pounds ground beef

Combine chili sauce and cranberries in a saucepan and heat for 5-10 minutes until like gravy. Mix onion and beef, roll into small balls. Drop rolled meatballs into mixture, cover and cook slowly for about 30-35 minutes.

Cheese Goodies

2 dozen.

¼ pound margarine
1¼ cups shredded sharp cheddar cheese
1 cup flour
½ teaspoon salt
¼ teaspoon pepper
¼ teaspoon paprika
2 cups Rice Krispies

Cream margarine and shredded cheese together. Add flour, salt, pepper and paprika. Fold in Rice Krispies. Form small balls and flatten with a spoon. Bake in preheated 350 degree oven for 12-15 minutes on ungreased cookie sheet.

Popcorn Mix

20 servings.

4 cups Cherrios
4 cups Kix
4 cups Crispix
14 cups popped popcorn
3 cups unsalted peanuts
½ pound butter
¾ cup Karo lite corn syrup
2 cups brown sugar, packed
2 teaspoons vanilla extract
½ teaspoon baking powder

In large bowl, mix the first 5 ingredients. Boil together butter, Karo syrup and brown sugar for 5 minutes. Turn off burner immediately. Add vanilla and baking powder. This will rise up high, so use large saucepan. Mix with cereal. Spray large roasting or lasagna pan with a non-stick vegetable spray and bake in 250 degree oven for 1 hour, stirring every 15 minutes.

Heavenly Ham

4 servings.

1 large round loaf French bread
16 ounces cream cheese
16 ounces sour cream
4 green onions, chopped (optional)
1 large can chopped Ortega chiles
½ pound chopped ham or chipped beef

Cut off top of French bread and scoop out the insides, making a bowl. Combine cream cheese, sour cream, green onions, chiles and ham. Fill the bread with the meat mixture and replace the top. Wrap in foil. Bake 1 hour at 350 degrees.

Wrap bread cubes taken from the inside of the loaf in foil and heat. Serve ham bowl with warmed bread cubes arranged around the base.

Chicken Wings

12 servings.

½ cup soy sauce
¼ cup sherry
1 clove garlic, minced
½ teaspoon cinnamon
½ cup brown sugar
½ teaspoon ginger
¼ teaspoon pepper
4-5 pounds chicken wings

Combine all ingredients except for chicken wings. Cut chicken wings in half, discarding wing tips. Pour ingredients over chicken wings and refrigerate overnight, stirring occasionally. Arrange chicken wings in shallow baking dish, cover with marinade. Bake in 350 degree oven for 1 hour.

Potato Things

8 servings.

12 small red potatoes
1 cup grated cheddar cheese
⅓ cup bacon bits
½ cup sour cream

Boil (or microwave) small potatoes until tender. Cut in half. With melon scoop remove small amount of potato. Top each potato half with approximately 1 teaspoon of grated cheese and a small amount of bacon bits. Bake in 350 degree oven for 15 minutes to melt cheese before serving. Place on tray with bowl of sour cream.

Zucchini Melts

6 servings.

6 medium size zucchini
2 tablespoons butter, softened
Salt
Pepper
3 tablespoons parmesan cheese

Slice zucchini in ¼″ slices. Arrange on cookie sheet. Butter, salt and pepper each slice. Sprinkle ½-1 teaspoon grated parmesan cheese on top of each. Slide under hot broiler for 1 minute or until cheese is melted. Arrange on dish and serve.

Smoked Salmon Log

10 to 12 servings.

1 pound can salmon, drained
1 8 ounce package light
cream cheese, softened
2 teaspoons prepared horseradish
¼ teaspoon liquid smoke
¼ teaspoon cayenne pepper
1 tablespoon lemon juice
1 tablespoon grated onion
3 tablespoons snipped parsley
½ cup chopped pecans

Flake salmon, removing skin and bones. Combine salmon, cream cheese, horseradish, liquid smoke, cayenne pepper, lemon juice and onion. Mix thoroughly. Chill several hours or overnight. Combine parsley and pecans in a shallow dish. Shape mixture into a log and roll in parsley-pecan mixture. Chill thoroughly. Serve with assorted crackers.

Herb Cream Cheese

2 cups.

2 8 ounce packages
cream cheese, softened
3 tablespoons milk or half and half
3 cloves garlic, minced
¼ cup dried dill or ½ cup fresh dill
¼ teaspoon pepper
1½ teaspoons dried chopped chives or
3 teaspoons fresh chives
12 drops hot pepper sauce
Crackers or sourdough baguettes, sliced

Blend first 7 ingredients together. Serve with crackers or baguettes. Recipe may be cut in half.

Muenster Cheese Pie

6 servings.

1 egg
¾ cup flour
½ teaspoon salt
⅛ teaspoon pepper
1 cup milk
1 cup shredded Muenster cheese

Combine egg, flour, salt, pepper and ½ cup milk in a small bowl. Beat until smooth. Add the remaining milk and beat until blended. Stir in ½ of the cheese. Pour into a well greased 8″ pie pan. Bake in 425 degree oven for 30 minutes. Sprinkle remaining cheese on top and bake until cheese is melted. Can be served as a main dish or appetizer.

Chutney Dip

10 to 12 servings.

8 ounces cream cheese
8 ounces cheddar cheese, grated
2 tablespoons sherry wine
1 teaspoon curry powder
1 6 ounce jar of chutney
3 scallions or green onions, chopped

Combine cream cheese, cheddar cheese, wine and curry powder. Place in serving dish. Top with chutney. Sprinkle with chopped scallions or green onion tops. Serve with crackers.

Salmon Dip

2 cups.

½ cup non-fat lemon or lime yogurt
¼ cup minced celery
3 tablespoons shallots, minced
Fresh dill
Pimiento
1 teaspoon lemon zest
1 tablespoon fresh lemon juice
¾ pound cooked salmon, flaked
6 drops tabasco
¼ teaspoon Beau Monde
¼ teaspoon lemon chili seasoning
4 heads Belgium endive

Blend together first 11 ingredients. Cover and refrigerate for 12-24 hours.

To serve, place in shallow bowl in center of plate. Surround with Belgium endive for dipping.

§ *Calories: 45 Fat: 1.6gm Cholesterol: 11 Sodium: 20mg*

Swiss Cheese Dip

2½ cups.

¼ cup mayonnaise
2 tablespoons chili sauce
1 cup cream-style cottage cheese
1 small wedge of onion
¼ teaspoon celery salt
1 cup cubed Swiss cheese
French bread, cubed

Place all ingredients except Swiss cheese and bread in the blender. Cover and process on high until smooth. Add cheese cubes gradually and process until smooth. Serve with toasted French bread cubes.

Horseradish Dip

2¼ cups.

3 tablespoons milk
2 cups creamed cottage cheese
2 tablespoons horseradish
½ teaspoon Worcestershire sauce
2 sprigs parsley

Place all ingredients in a blender and process on high until smooth. Serve with fresh fruit or vegetables.

§ *Calories: 26 Fat: 1.1gm Cholesterol: 4mg Sodium: 99mg*

Skinny Dip

1½ cups.

1 container firm tofu
2 tablespoons horseradish
4 tablespoons dried dill weed
1 tablespoon Dijon mustard
1 small bunch scallions, finely chopped
1 tablespoon lemon juice
2 tablespoons prepared low-calorie ranch dressing
White pepper to taste

Drain tofu. Leave in strainer for about 1 hour. Place tofu and all the rest of the ingredients in food processor bowl and process until smooth. Make at least a few hours ahead to let flavors blend.

Use as a dip for veggies or for a spread on crackers.

§ *Calories: 27 Fat: 1.1gm Cholesterol: 0mg Sodium: 67mg*

Low-Cal Spread

1 cup.

1 6 ounce can water packed tuna,
rinsed and drained
1 small can water chestnuts, drained
1 bunch green onions, finely chopped
2 tablespoons lemon juice
Few drops hot pepper sauce
1 teaspoon dried or
fresh dill (optional)
4 tablespoons low-calorie
Italian dressing

Place all ingredients in food processor. Process until smooth. Serve with crackers.

§ *Calories: 26 Fat: 0.1gm Cholesterol: 0mg Sodium: 80mg*

Tortilla Roll Ups

20 servings.

1 8 ounce package cream cheese
5 tablespoons Dijon mustard
12 flour tortillas
Spinach or basil leaves
12 thin slices Muenster cheese
12 thin slices roast beef or ham

Mix together cream cheese and mustard until creamy. Spread mixture on tortillas. Cover mixture with spinach or basil leaves. Cut cheese slices to fit and place on top of spinach leaves. Cut roast beef or ham to fit and place on top of cheese. Roll tortillas carefully and wrap in a wet dish towel for at least 1 hour or overnight. Slice carefully when ready to serve. Spear each with toothpick.

Marinated Raw Vegetables

36 servings.

2 heads cauliflower
3 green peppers
2 pounds small carrots
1 bunch celery
1 bunch broccoli
2 cucumbers
1 pound fresh mushrooms
4 zucchini
½ cup salad oil
½ cup olive oil
½ cup white wine vinegar
½-¾ cup sugar
3 cloves garlic, minced
1 tablespoon salt
1 tablespoon prepared mustard
2 teaspoons tarragon leaves
Pepper to taste
18 cherry tomatoes
4 tablespoons chives, minced
1 large solid tomato
1 bunch watercress

Cut up the first 8 ingredients into bite-size pieces. Combine the salad oil, olive oil and vinegar. Add the sugar, garlic, salt, mustard, tarragon and pepper. Pour the mixture over the vegetables. Cover and chill for at least 12 hours or overnight. Stir occasionally.

To serve, arrange the vegetables on a platter. Garnish with cherry tomatoes and sprinkle top with the minced chives. For additional garnish, use the peel of a large tomato to form a rose, and place on the watercress in the center of the vegetable platter.

Cheese Roll

20 servings.

1 pound velveeta cheese
1 4 ounce can Ortega diced green chiles
2 8 ounce packages cream cheese
1 1.75 ounce package garlic dip mix
1 1.75 ounce package green onion dip mix or
½ package onion soup mix
Bacon bits to taste
Parsley

Place velveeta cheese bar between 2 large sheets of waxed paper. Plastic will not work. With rolling pin, roll into an oblong shape as thin as possible.

Make a mixture of all other ingredients and spread over cheese. Then trim edges. With hands underneath waxed paper, begin to roll cheese into a "jellyroll" form. Garnish with parsley and serve with crispies of any kind.

Pickled Shrimp

6 servings.

1 cup cider vinegar
2 teaspoons dry mustard
½ cup tomato sauce
1½ cups olive oil
2 tablespoons tabasco sauce
2 tablespoons Worcestershire sauce
1 teaspoon salt
½ teaspoon pepper
3 tablespoons capers
1 onion
2 cups red onions, sliced
1 cup bell peppers, sliced
2½-3 pounds large shrimp (12 per pound), cooked, peeled and deveined

In large non-metallic container, combine vinegar, mustard, tomato sauce, oil, Worcestershire sauce, tabasco, salt and pepper. Blend thoroughly.

Layer capers, pepper slices, onion rings and shrimp in container. Cover with marinade and seal tightly and refrigerate. Stir occasionally. Drain liquid and transfer to a serving dish. Serve with crackers or French bread pieces. Prepare 2-3 days ahead for best flavor.

Hot Mulled Cranberry Orange Cup

5 cups.

2 cups cranberry juice cocktail
⅓ cup sugar
8 whole cloves
1 2″ cinnamon stick
Peel from 1 orange, cut into strips
3 cups orange juice
Cinnamon sticks (optional)

In 2 quart saucepan, stir together cranberry juice, sugar, cloves, cinnamon stick and orange peel. Bring to a boil. Reduce heat and simmer 10 minutes; strain. Stir in orange juice. Heat through but do not boil. Serve hot. Garnish with cinnamon sticks if desired.

Wassil

10 to 12 servings.

Juice of 6 oranges
Juice of 4 lemons
2½ cups sugar
1 teaspoon ginger
3 sticks cinnamon
2 teaspoons cloves
2 cups strong tea
1 quart cider
2 cups hot water
Brandy (optional)

Combine fruit juices, sugar and spices to make a thick syrup. Add remaining ingredients and let stand overnight. Serve hot. Brandy may be added if desired.

Hot Spiced Cider

2 quarts.

½ cup brown sugar
1 tablespoon whole cloves (12 or more)
½ teaspoon allspice (8 whole)
3 sticks cinnamon
Dash of salt
Dash of nutmeg
2 quarts apple cider
1 tablespoon lemon juice (optional)

Combine all ingredients in a 3 quart saucepan. Bring to a boil, stirring constantly. Cover and simmer for 20 minutes. Strain to remove spices. Serve hot in punch cups. May use cinnamon sticks for stirrers.

Perfect Punch

2½ gallons.

1½ cups sugar
6 cups water
1 12 ounce can frozen orange juice, thawed
1 46 ounce can pineapple-grapefruit juice
5 bananas
2 1 liter bottles 7-up

In a large kettle or bowl, stir sugar in water until dissolved. Add orange juice, undiluted, and pineapple-grapefruit juice. Pour some of this mixture into blender, add bananas and puree until smooth. Add banana mixture back into juice mixture. Stir until blended. Pour into two 1 gallon ziplock freezer bags. Freeze.

Three hours before serving, remove bags from freezer to partially thaw. In a serving bowl, mix 1 bag of frozen mix and 1 bottle of 7-up. Stir until blended.

Chocolate Eggnog

1 quart.

3 cups dairy eggnog, chilled
1 cup chocolate milk
½ cup creme de cacao
1 cup whipping cream
Shaved chocolate

In a pitcher, combine eggnog, chocolate milk and creme de cacao. Cover and chill. Just before serving, whip cream to soft peaks. Garnish each serving with a dollop of the whipped cream and some of the shaved chocolate.

Egg Nog

5 pints.

6 eggs, separated
¾ cup sugar
1 pint cream
1 pint half and half
1 pint Four Roses
1 ounce rum
Grated nutmeg

Separately beat the yolks and whites of eggs. Add ½ cup sugar to yolks while beating. Add ¼ cup sugar to whites after they have been beaten very stiff. Mix egg whites with yolks. Stir in cream and half and half. Add Four Roses and rum. Blend thoroughly. Serve very cold with grated nutmeg.

Non-Alcoholic Coffee Liquor

8 to 10 servings.

6 ounces water
10 heaping teaspoons instant coffee
2 tablespoons sugar
6 ounces corn syrup
2 teaspoons vanilla extract

Bring the water to a boil in a small pan. While it is boiling, stir vigorously and slowly add coffee, then sugar. Be sure both are completely dissolved, then add syrup. Partially cool, add vanilla and stir. Cool. Great for a topping on vanilla ice cream!

Tropical Tea Mix

4½ to 5 cups.

2 cups Tang
1 3 ounce package powdered
lemonade mix
¾ cup instant tea
1⅓ cups sugar
1 teaspoon cinnamon
¼ teaspoon cloves

Mix all ingredients and store in airtight container. Use 2 tablespoons per cup of boiling water.

Orange Frost

2 to 4 servings.

1½ cups fresh orange juice
½ teaspoon honey
3 tablespoons dry nonfat milk
½ teaspoon grated orange rind
3 ice cubes
Mint sprigs

Combine all ingredients except the mint sprigs. Blend or shake until frothy. Serve in a chilled glass with mint sprig garnish.

Kahlua

1 quart.

3 cups sugar
9 teaspoons instant coffee
4 cups water
2½ cups vodka
3 teaspoons vanilla extract

Combine sugar, instant coffee and water in saucepan. Simmer for 1 hour. Cool. Add vodka and vanilla. Pour into sterilized bottles or jars. Can be kept in cool place.

Fruit Champagne Punch

25 servings.

1 basket strawberries
¼ cup sugar
Juice of 1 lemon
¼ cup brandy
1 fifth white wine
1 fifth champagne
1 28 ounce bottle soda
1 orange, thinly sliced

Wash, hull and slice strawberries. Combine berries, sugar, lemon juice, brandy and 1 cup white wine and chill at least 2 hours. Stir remaining wine into mixture.

Place ice ring in punch bowl and pour berry mixture over ice. Add chilled champagne and soda. Garnish with whole strawberries and sliced oranges.

Rum Punch

30 punch cups.

¾ pound lump sugar
2 quarts water
1 quart lemon juice
2 fifths light rum
1 fifth California brandy
½ cup peach brandy

Dissolve lump sugar in water. Add remaining ingredients. Cool at least 2 hours before serving.

Lemon Sangria

1½ quarts.

3½ cups dry white wine, chilled
3 unpeeled lemons, sliced
1 unpeeled orange, sliced
1 green apple, peeled, cored and
cut into wedges
Small bunches green grapes (optional)
½ cup Cognac
¼ cup sugar
1 10 ounce bottle club soda, chilled
Ice cubes

Combine all ingredients except soda and ice cubes in large pitcher and chill overnight. Just before serving, add soda and ice cubes and stir lightly. Pour into glasses, adding fruit if desired.

Peach Margaritas

4 servings.

6 ounces gold tequila
3 ounces Triple Sec
2 tablespoons lime juice
4 teaspoons sugar
2 cups sliced fresh peaches or
2 cups canned sliced peaches, drained
8 ice cubes

Combine tequila, Triple Sec, lime juice, sugar, peaches and ice cubes in blender. Blend until peaches are pureed. Serve in sugar-rimmed glasses or salt-rimmed if preferred.

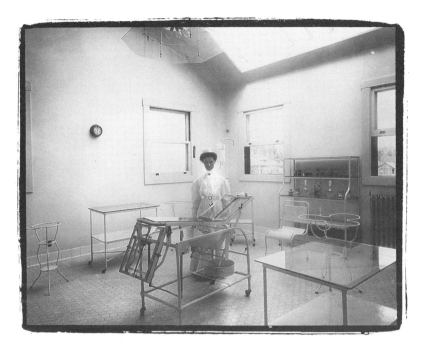

The "complete and convenient operating room" of 1907

breads

Homemade Yeast

Boil six large potatoes in three pints of water. Tie a handful of hops in a small muslin bag and boil with the potatoes; when thoroughly cooked drain the water on enough flour to make a thin batter; set this on the stove or range and scald it enough to cook the flour (this makes the yeast keep longer); remove it from the fire and when cool enough, add the potatoes mashed, also half a cup of sugar, half a tablespoonful of ginger, two of salt and a teacupful of yeast. Let it stand in a warm place, until it has thoroughly risen, then put it in a large mouthed jug and cork tightly; set away in a cool place.

The jug should be scalded before putting in the yeast. Two-thirds of a coffee-cupful of this yeast will make four loaves.

The White House Cookbook © 1887

Orange Cranberry Bread

1 loaf.

½ cup slivered orange peel
1 cup sugar
¼ cup water
¼ cup butter or margarine
1 cup orange juice
2 eggs, beaten
2½ cups sifted flour
1 tablespoon baking powder
½ teaspoon baking soda
½ teaspoon salt
¼ cup wheat germ or finely chopped nuts
1 cup coarsely chopped fresh cranberries

Prepare orange peel; grate or finely slice. Combine sugar and water in saucepan. Add peel and cook, stirring constantly until sugar dissolves. Cook over low heat for another 5 minutes, continuing to stir. Remove from heat. Add butter and stir until melted. Cool slightly. Add orange juice and eggs. Blend well.

Sift together flour, baking powder, soda and salt. Stir in wheat. Add liquid until flour is moistened. Stir in cranberries. Pour mixture into a greased and floured 9″ x 5″ loaf pan. Bake in 350 degree oven for 1 hour. Cool 10 minutes. Remove from pan and cool completely.

Corn Bread

10 to 12 servings.

2 cups Bisquick or baking mix
½ teaspoon baking soda
1 cup yellow cornmeal
¾ cup sugar
½ cup melted butter
1 cup buttermilk
2 eggs, slightly beaten
1 8.5 ounce can creamed sweet corn

Preheat oven to 350 degrees. Grease 13″ x 9″ x 2″ baking dish or pan.

Combine Bisquick, baking soda, cornmeal and sugar. Add melted butter, buttermilk, eggs and creamed sweet corn. Mix well. Batter will be lumpy. Pour into greased pan and bake for 20-30 minutes.

Banana Nut Bread

1 loaf.

½ cup butter or margarine, softened
1 cup sugar
2 eggs
1 cup mashed bananas (about 2)
1½ tablespoons milk
1 tablespoon fresh lemon juice
2 cups all-purpose flour
1½ teaspoons baking powder
½ teaspoon baking soda
¼ teaspoon salt
1 cup chopped walnuts

Cream butter and sugar. Beat in eggs one at a time. Mix bananas, milk and lemon juice, combine with first mixture. Sift flour with baking powder, soda and salt, add to mixture. Add nuts and bake in greased 9″ x 5″ x 3″ loaf pan in 350 degree oven for 1 hour 5 minutes-1 hour 10 minutes or until toothpick inserted in center comes out clean.

Zucchini Oatbran Bread

2 loaves.

¾ cup egg beaters
1 cup corn or safflower oil
2 cups sugar
2 cups grated zucchini
1 teaspoon vanilla extract
1 cup oatbran
1 cup wheat flour
1 cup white flour
1 teaspoon salt (optional)
1 teaspoon baking soda
2 teaspoons cinnamon
1 teaspoon baking powder

Spray two 9″ x 5″ x 3″ loaf pans with a low fat vegetable spray. Whip egg beaters slightly, add oil, sugar, zucchini and vanilla. Sift dry ingredients together. Add to egg mixture. Blend well. Divide evenly between 2 loaf pans. Bake in 350 degree oven for 1 hour or until done.

Wry Braid

2 braids.

2 packages active dry yeast
2 cups warm water
(not hot-should be 110-115 degrees)
1 envelope onion soup mix
⅓ cup sugar
2 tablespoons molasses
1 teaspoon salt
1 egg
⅓ cup shortening, softened
6-6½ cups flour (not self-rising)

In a mixing bowl, dissolve yeast in warm water. Add soup mix, and stir to dissolve completely. Add remaining ingredients and one half of the flour; beat with spoon until smooth. Mix in enough remaining flour until dough handles easily. Turn onto lightly floured board. Knead until smooth (about 10 minutes). Place in greased bowl, turning once to bring greased side up. Cover with cloth; let rise in a warm place (85 degrees) until double, about 1 hour.

Punch down, cover and let rise until almost double, about 30 minutes. Divide dough in half. Divide each half into 3 equal parts and roll into 14″ strands. Place on greased baking sheet, braid loosely, fasten ends and tuck under securely. Brush with butter, cover with cloth; let rise until double, about 40-50 minutes. Bake braids in 375 degree oven for 25-30 minutes.

Carrot Bread

1 loaf.

3 medium carrots, grated
1⅓ cups sugar
1⅓ cups water
1 cup raisins
2 tablespoons margarine
1 teaspoon ground cloves
1 teaspoon cinnamon
1 teaspoon nutmeg
1 cup walnuts, chopped
2 cups flour
2 teaspoons baking soda
Pinch of salt

Place grated carrots in saucepan. Add sugar, water, raisins, margarine, cloves, cinnamon and nutmeg. Bring to boil, reduce heat and simmer at a low boil for 5 minutes. Remove from heat and allow to become cold.

Mix walnuts, flour, soda and salt and add to above mixture. Place in greased loaf pan and bake in 325 degree oven for 1 hour 15 minutes-1 hour 30 minutes.

Bubble Loaf

1 loaf.

½ cup chopped pecans
1 package parker house frozen rolls, defrosted
1 6 ounce package vanilla or butterscotch pudding mix (non-instant)
¾ cup brown sugar
1 teaspoon cinnamon
6 tablespoons butter

Grease a 9″ bundt pan well. Sprinkle nuts on bottom. Cut each parker house roll into thirds. Place rolls in pan. Combine pudding mix, brown sugar and cinnamon together and sprinkle over rolls. Let rise. Cut 6 tablespoons butter over top of dough. Bake in 350 degree oven for 30-35 minutes. Turn upside down when baked so syrup will run over rolls.

Chile Cornbread

6 servings.

1 cup flour, sifted
½ teaspoon salt
1 tablespoon baking powder
1 tablespoon sugar
1 cup cornmeal
2 eggs, beaten
1 cup milk
¼ cup oil
8 ounces whole kernel corn
½ cup canned chopped chiles

Sift together flour, salt, baking powder and sugar. Stir in cornmeal. Combine eggs, milk and oil and add to dry ingredients, mixing just to dampen flour. Drain corn and fold into batter with chiles. Turn into well greased 8″ square baking pan or muffin pan. Bake in 425 oven for 30 minutes. Serve hot with butter.

Grandma's Lemon Bread

1 loaf.

6 tablespoons butter
1 cup sugar
2 eggs
½ cup milk
1½ cups flour
1 teaspoon baking powder
½ teaspoon salt
Grated rind of 1 large lemon
Juice from 1 large lemon
½ cup sugar

Cream butter and sugar and beat in eggs. Add milk and mix well. Sift dry ingredients together and add to batter. Add lemon rind. Place in greased 4″ x 8″ loaf pan and bake in preheated 350 degree oven for 1 hour.

While bread is baking, mix juice of 1 lemon and ½ cup sugar together. Spoon glaze over hot bread before removing from pan. Use all of the glaze.

Picnic Pear Nut Bread

1 loaf.

2 fresh bartlett pears, fully ripe
2 large eggs, beaten
1 cup whole bran
1½ cups sifted all-purpose flour
½ cup sugar
1 teaspoon baking powder
½ teaspoon salt
½ teaspoon baking soda
¼ cup shortening, softened
½ cup chopped walnuts

Lemon Mint Butter:
1 cup butter or margarine, softened
1 teaspoon grated lemon peel
2 tablespoons chopped
fresh mint leaves

Core and finely chop unpeeled pears to measure 1¼ cups. Combine with eggs and bran; let stand while preparing remaining ingredients.

Sift flour with sugar, baking powder, salt and soda into mixing bowl. Add shortening and pear-bran mixture; mix until all of flour is moistened. Stir in walnuts. Turn into a well-greased 8½" x 4½" x 2½" loaf pan. Let stand 20 minutes. Bake in 350 degree oven about 1 hour or until toothpick inserted in center comes out clean and dry. Let stand 10 minutes, then turn out onto wire rack to cool. If desired, spread with Lemon-Mint Butter.

Lemon Mint Butter:
Beat butter with lemon peel and 2 tablespoons fresh mint leaves.

Pineapple Coconut Bread

3 loaves.

1 20 ounce can crushed pineapple
1 10 ounce package moist coconut
4 eggs
½ cup sugar
4 cups flour
2 teaspoons salt
2 teaspoons baking soda

Mix all ingredients together and pour into 3 greased 9" x 5" loaf pans. Bake in 325 degree oven for 1 hour. Bread freezes well.

Party Cheese Bread

12 servings.

**Medium sized round loaf
of sourdough bread
¼ pound sweet butter
1 3 ounce package cream cheese
½ cup grated cheddar cheese, packed
2 egg whites**

Cut crust from bread and slice into finger-sized pieces approximately 1½″ x ½″. In double boiler or microwave melt butter, cream cheese and cheddar cheese. After mixture is smooth, cool slightly and then fold in stiffly beaten egg whites. Using a fork, dip bread fingers into mixture. Shake off excess. Place coated bread on greased cookie sheet. Refrigerate overnight.

Preheat oven to 375 degrees. Bake for 13-15 minutes or until golden brown.

Irish Soda Bread

2 loaves.

**4 cups sifted all-purpose flour
1 tablespoon baking powder
2 teaspoons salt
1 teaspoon baking soda
¼ cup butter
¼ cup sugar
1½ cups raisins
1 teaspoon caraway seeds (optional)
1 egg, well beaten
1¾ cups buttermilk**

Sift flour, baking powder, salt and soda together into a large bowl. Add butter and work with hands, until mixture resembles fine crumbs. Add sugar, raisins and caraway seeds. Mix well. Combine egg and buttermilk and add to dry ingredients. Stir with spoon, then turn out on a floured surface and knead 2-3 minutes until smooth. Divide dough in half and shape into two round loaves. Place on large, ungreased baking sheet. Cut a deep cross in top of each loaf. Bake in 375 degree oven for 40-45 minutes.

Oatmeal Tea Bread

1 loaf.

1¼ cups flour
1 cup quick rolled oats
¾ cup sugar
1 teaspoon salt, scant
1 teaspoon baking powder
1 teaspoon baking soda
½ teaspoon cinnamon
½ teaspoon nutmeg
2 large eggs
1¼ cups applesauce or
persimmon puree
½ cup raisins
⅓ cup vegetable oil
¼ cup milk

Topping:
2 tablespoons brown sugar,
firmly packed
2 tablespoons chopped pecans
¼ teaspoon cinnamon

Preheat oven to 350 degrees. Mix flour, oats, sugar, salt, baking powder, baking soda, cinnamon and nutmeg together in large bowl. Set aside. Combine eggs, applesauce, raisins, oil and milk in bowl. Make a well in reserved flour mixture. Pour applesauce mixture into well and combine by hand until flour is just moistened. Grease a 9″ x 5″ x 3″ loaf pan and turn batter into pan.

Topping:
Mix brown sugar, pecans and cinnamon together in small bowl. Sprinkle on top of batter. Bake in 350 degree oven for 55 minutes to 1 hour, or until toothpick inserted in middle comes out clean. Cool in pan 10 minutes. Remove from pan and cool on rack.

Orange Bread

2 loaves.

4 medium oranges (1 cup cooked peel)
1½ cups sugar
2 cups sifted flour
¼ teaspoon salt
2 teaspoons baking powder
½ cup milk
1 egg, beaten
½ cup orange water

Cut oranges into quarters. Place in a medium pot, cover with cold water. Cook 20 minutes; drain, saving ½ cup of the orange water. Cook 20 minutes more in fresh water. Drain. Remove the meat of the orange and some of the white off the peel. Slice the peel into fine pieces. Cook in 1 cup sugar until blended. Cool. Set aside.

Combine flour, salt, baking powder and ½ cup sugar in bowl. In a separate bowl combine milk, egg and ½ cup orange water. Add to dry ingredients, mix well. Add peel, blend thoroughly.

Preheat oven to 350 degrees. Bake in two greased loaf pans, 7½″ x 4″, for 1 hour. Recipe can be doubled. Freezes well.

Applesauce Nut Bread

1 loaf.

2 cups flour
¾ cup sugar
3 teaspoons baking powder
½ teaspoon baking soda
½ teaspoon cinnamon
1 cup chopped nuts
1 egg, beaten
1 cup applesauce
2 tablespoons oil

Mix flour, sugar, baking powder, soda and cinnamon with a fork. Stir in nuts and set aside. Lightly combine egg, applesauce and oil. Add to dry ingredients and stir until blended. Pour into greased 9″ x 5″ x 3″ loaf pan. Bake in 350 degree oven for 50 minutes or until toothpick inserted in center of bread comes out clean.

Santa's Bread

2 loaves.

½ cup margarine
1 cup sugar
2 eggs
1 teaspoon vanilla extract
2 cups flour
1 teaspoon baking soda
Pinch of salt
1 cup mashed bananas
1 11 ounce can mandarin orange
segments, drained
1 6 ounce package chocolate chips
1 cup shredded coconut
⅔ cup sliced almonds or walnuts
½ cup chopped maraschino cherries
½ cup chopped dates or figs
Powdered sugar

Preheat oven to 350 degrees. Cream margarine with sugar. Add eggs and vanilla; beat until fluffy. Sift flour with baking soda and salt; add to butter alternately with bananas. Stir in oranges, chocolate chips, coconut, ½ cup almonds, cherries and dates.

Pour batter into two greased 7½″ x 3¾″ loaf pans. Sprinkle remaining sliced almonds over top. Bake 1 hour 15 minutes. When loaf is done, sprinkle powdered sugar over top.

Banana Nut Muffins

12 muffins.

2¼ cups oat bran
1 tablespoon baking powder
¼ cup brown sugar
¼ cup chopped walnuts or pecans
1¼ cups skim milk
2 bananas, very ripe
2 egg whites
2 tablespoons vegetable oil

Preheat oven to 425 degrees. Mix the dry ingredients in a bowl. Mix the milk, bananas, egg whites, and oil in a bowl or blender. Add the dry ingredients and mix. Line the muffin pan with paper baking cups and fill with batter. Bake for 17 minutes.

§ *Calories: 120 Fat: 5.1gm Cholesterol: 1mg Sodium: 98mg*

Philadelphia Cinnamon Buns

6 servings.

1 loaf frozen bread dough
½ cup Karo dark corn syrup
1 cup raisins
½ cup butter or margarine, softened
½ cup brown sugar
Cinnamon to taste

Defrost dough. Butter 2 pie plates or cake pans thoroughly. Spread Karo dark syrup over bottom of pans and then top each with ¼ cup of raisins. Using half of the dough, roll into a rectangle about 12″ x 6″. Spread with softened butter. Add half of the brown sugar and cinnamon. Sprinkle on half of the remaining raisins. Roll in jellyroll fashion lengthwise. Cut into 6 individual buns. Put into prepared pan. Repeat for the other half of dough.

Cover with towel and let rise for about 5 hours. Bake in 350 degree oven for 20 minutes. Immediately after removing from oven, turn baking dish upside down on serving platter.

Raisin Bran Muffins

3½ dozen.

4 eggs, beaten
1 cup oil
1 quart buttermilk
3 cups sugar
5 cups flour
5 teaspoons baking soda
2 teaspoons salt
1 15 ounce package Raisin Bran cereal

Combine eggs, oil and buttermilk. Mix together all dry ingredients in a large bowl. Add the egg mixture. Mix and store in the refrigerator overnight before using. Lightly grease muffin tins and scoop batter into tins. Bake in 400 degree oven for 15-20 minutes.

Note: Do not stir batter before filling muffin tins.

Cheese Scones

15 scones.

8 ounces Bisquick
1 teaspoon mustard powder
½ teaspoon salt
Pinch of salt
2 ounces butter
4 ounces grated cheddar cheese
1 egg, beaten
4 tablespoons milk
Beaten egg or milk to glaze

Sift Bisquick, mustard powder, salt and pepper into a bowl. Cut in butter with a pastry blender or fork until the mixture resembles fine butter crumbs. Stir in 3 ounces of the cheese. Add egg and sufficient milk to mix into a soft dough.

Knead very lightly on a floured board and roll out dough ¾" thick. Cut into rounds 1½"-2" across and place close together on a greased baking sheet. Brush with beaten egg or milk and sprinkle with the remaining cheese. Bake for 20 minutes in pre-heated 400 degree oven.

Caramel Orange Rolls

12 rolls.

¼ cup sugar
1 teaspoon grated orange rind
1½ tablespoons orange juice
¼ teaspoon mace
1 tablespoon margarine
12 brown and serve rolls

Combine sugar, orange rind, orange juice, mace and margarine. Spread over bottom of ungreased shallow pan. Place rolls upside down over sugar mixture. Bake in 400 degree oven for 15 minutes.

Remove from oven. Let rolls stand in pan until syrup thickens, or about 1 minute. Invert pan and remove rolls so that the caramel orange topping coats rolls.

Corn Muffin Surprise

12 muffins.

1 medium ear of corn
16 tablespoons unsalted butter
(8 ounces)
3 small jalapeno peppers,
finely chopped
2 teaspoons fresh chopped rosemary
2 tablespoons light brown sugar,
packed
1 egg
1 teaspoon salt
1 teaspoon baking soda
1 cup all-purpose flour
1 cup stoneground cornmeal
1¼ cups buttermilk

Preheat the oven to 425 degrees. Cut the kernels from the ear of corn. Set aside.

In a saucepan, melt 1½ tablespoons of butter. Brush medium-size muffin tins with some of the melted butter and set aside. Add the jalapeno peppers to the remaining butter in the pan and cook slowly for 1 minute. Remove from the heat. Add the corn and rosemary to the pan with the peppers and set aside.

In the bowl of an electric mixer, cream the remaining butter with the sugar, then add the egg and mix well. Scrape down the sides of the bowl as necessary. The mixture should be light and fluffy.

Mix together the salt, baking soda, flour and cornmeal. To the butter add a quarter of the flour mixture, then a quarter of the buttermilk, mixing well after each addition. Continue with alternate additions of flour and buttermilk until all has been used. Stir in the jalapeno and corn mixture.

Spoon the batter into the muffin tins until they are three-quarters full and bake for 18-20 minutes. A toothpick inserted in the center will come out clean.

Let the muffins cool for about 5 minutes and then remove from the tins.

Lemon Muffins

1½ dozen.

1¾ cups flour
¾ cup sugar
1 tablespoon baking powder
1 teaspoon salt
1 egg
⅔ cup milk
Grated lemon peel from 2 lemons
1 tablespoon lemon juice
⅓ cup oil

Mix together flour, ½ cup sugar, baking powder, and salt. Beat egg lightly in separate bowl. Stir in milk, grated peel from 1 lemon, lemon juice and oil. Add to flour mixture. Stir until moistened. Fill each muffin cup two-thirds full. Sprinkle tops of muffins with remaining sugar and lemon peel. Bake in 400 degree oven for 20 minutes.

Melt-in-Your-Mouth Pancakes

4 servings.

4 eggs, separated
1 cup sour cream
1 cup small curd cottage cheese
¾ cup flour, sifted
¼ teaspoon salt
1 tablespoon sugar

Beat egg whites until stiff and set aside. Beat egg yolks until creamy. To egg yolks, add sour cream and cottage cheese. Blend thoroughly. Resift flour with dry ingredients and add to cottage cheese mixture. Gently fold in egg whites.

Heat a lightly buttered griddle. Drop batter by spoonfuls and cook until bubbly, turn and brown other side. Serve with melted butter and warm syrup.

French Fruit Toast

4 servings.

4 slices thick white bread
½ cup milk
2 eggs beaten
¼ cup butter or margarine
½ cup favorite jam
1 cup whole milk ricotta cheese
Variety of fresh fruits (sliced peaches, sliced pears or raspberries)
2 tablespoons butter
¼ cup sour cream

Dip both sides of bread into milk and then into beaten egg. Fry both sides in butter until brown on edges. Remove toast and spread with jam. Top with ricotta cheese. Saute fruit in 2 tablespoons butter briefly and place on top of each piece of toast. Top with dollop of sour cream and serve warm.

Easy Coffee Cake

8 servings.

½ cup butter
1 cup sugar
2 eggs
2 cups sifted flour
2 teaspoons baking powder
Dash salt
1 5 ounce can evaporated milk
Cinnamon
Sugar
½ cup raisins, optional
Nuts, chopped

Cream butter and sugar. Add eggs. Combine flour, baking powder and salt. Add flour mixture alternately with milk. Pour half of the batter into 8" x 8" pan. Sprinkle with cinnamon and sugar. Add raisins if desired. Pour remaining batter in and sprinkle with additional cinnamon and sugar and chopped nuts. Bake at 350 degrees for 1 hour.

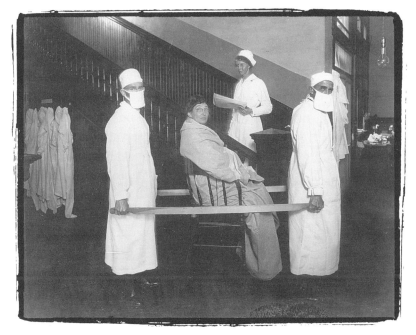

Patient transport, circa 1909

casseroles

Veal Olives

Cut up slice of veal, about half an inch thick, into squares of three inches. Mix up a little salt pork, chopped with bread crumbs, one onion, a little pepper, salt, sweet marjoram, and one egg well beaten; put this mixture upon the piece of veal, fastening the four corners together with little bird skewers; lay them in a pan with sufficient veal gravy or light stock to cover the bottom of the pan, dredge with flour and set in a hot oven. When browned on top, put a small bit of butter on each, and let them remain until quite tender, which will take twenty minutes.

Serve with horse-radish.

The White House Cookbook © 1887

Layered Tortillas

4 servings.

6 tablespoons vegetable oil
4 8" flour tortillas
¼ cup chopped green onion
⅓ cup mild taco sauce
4 ounce can chopped green chiles, drained
8 ounce can fried beans
1 cup shredded Monterey Jack cheese
½ cup shredded cheddar cheese
Iceberg lettuce, shredded
Tomatoes, chopped

Heat oven to 375 degrees. In 10" skillet, heat 4 tablespoons oil.

Fry tortillas for 5-10 seconds on each side until lightly browned. Drain well on paper towels. Add remaining 2 tablespoons oil to skillet. Saute onion and stir in taco sauce and green chiles.

Place 1 tortilla on ungreased cookie sheet. Top with one-third of the beans, one-third of the onion mixture and one-third of the Monterey Jack cheese. Repeat layering 2 more times ending with tortilla on top. Sprinkle with cheddar cheese.

Bake at 375 degrees for 15-20 minutes or until cheese is melted. Place on serving platter and top with lettuce and tomatoes. Cut into wedges to serve.

All American Macaroni & Cheese

10 servings.

1 pound macaroni
2 pounds sharp cheddar cheese, grated
1½ pints sour cream
Salt and pepper to taste

Cook macaroni. Mix grated cheese and sour cream with cooked macaroni. Add salt and pepper to taste. Place in a 9" x 13" casserole and bake in 350 degree oven for 45 minutes.

Fondue Monterey

12 servings.

12 slices egg bread
¼ pound butter
1 12 ounce can whole
kernel corn, drained
1 7 ounce can Ortega chiles diced
3 cups grated Monterey Jack cheese
4 eggs, slightly beaten
3 cups milk
Salt to taste

Trim crust from bread. Spread with butter and cut each slice in half. Arrange half the bread slices in a 9″ x 13″ buttered dish. Layer with half the corn. Arrange one half of the chiles over corn and sprinkle with one half of grated cheese. Repeat layers.

Combine eggs, milk and salt and pour over entire casserole. Cover and refrigerate four hours or longer (best if done overnight). Bake in 350 degree oven for 50 minutes uncovered.

Spinach Noodle Ring

6 servings.

1 8 ounce package wide noodles,
cooked and drained
½ pint sour cream
2 packages dry onion soup mix
1 stick melted margarine
5 eggs, beaten
1 10 ounce package chopped
leaf spinach

Combine all ingredients together, except spinach. Mix thoroughly and set aside. Cook spinach and drain very well. Mix with noodle mixture. Place in greased ring mold. Bake at 350 degrees for 1 hour. Decorate with cooked carrots in center of mold if desired.

Nuv's Green Noodle Casserole

6 servings.

½ pound spinach noodles
2 teaspoons chopped onions
½ pound sliced mushrooms
2 tablespoons butter
2 cans cream of mushroom soup
2 7 ounce cans chopped clams
1 small carton sour cream
¾ cup white wine
2 teaspoons curry
2 teaspoons fresh chopped parsley
Salt and pepper
Grated cheese (optional)

Cook noodles. Saute onions and mushrooms in butter. Combine with all other ingredients except noodles and grated cheese.

Put half of noodles in well-buttered 9" x 13" casserole. Cover with sauce. Top with remainder of noodles. Cover with aluminum foil and bake 45 minutes in 350 degree oven. Sprinkle with grated cheese if desired.

Breakfast Custard

8 to 10 servings.

1 loaf cinnamon raisin bread, crust removed and sliced
4 ounce butter, melted
7 eggs
3 egg yolks
¾ cup sugar
1 cup heavy cream
3 cups milk
1 teaspoon vanilla extract
Powdered sugar

Arrange one-third of the bread in the bottom of a 9" x 13" baking dish. Coat with melted butter. Continue to layer bread and coat with butter two more times. Combine remaining ingredients except powdered sugar, blend thoroughly. Pour mixture over bread.

Set dish in larger pan. Fill larger pan with hot water. Bake in 350 degree oven for 1 hour. Let stand 20 minutes before serving. Sprinkle with powdered sugar.

Sausage-Egg Casserole

6 servings.

1 pound mild bulk sausage
6 eggs
2 cups milk
1 teaspoon salt
1 teaspoon mustard
6 slices white bread, crusts removed and cubed
1 cup grated cheddar cheese
1 green pepper, chopped
1 can mushrooms, drained

Brown sausage, drain off fat. Cool and crumble, set aside. In mixing bowl, beat eggs; add milk, salt and mustard. Add bread cubes, cheese, sausage, green pepper and mushrooms. Stir just until blended. Put into a greased baking dish or casserole. Refrigerate overnight. Bake 45 minutes at 350 degrees or until high, puffed and brown.

Brunch Casserole

10 servings.

½ pound grated Monterey Jack cheese
2 cups cottage cheese
½ cup parmesan cheese
½ bunch chopped spinach
1 teaspoon salt
½ chopped onion
¼ teaspoon mint
½ cup chopped parsley
4 ounces sliced mushrooms
1 egg
½ package filo dough
½ pound melted unsalted butter

Combine all the ingredients except the filo dough and butter. Coat a 9" x 13" casserole pan with a non-stick vegetable spray.

Layer 6 sheets of filo into pan, buttering every other one. Add ½ of cheese mixture. Layer 4 sheets of filo dough on top, buttering every other. Add rest of mixture. Top with 6 sheets of filo dough, buttering every other. Cut casserole in 10 portions (more if smaller portions are desired). Bake, uncovered, in 350 degree oven about 45 minutes or until browned. Also good reheated.

Filo Cheese Casserole

9 to 12 servings.

1 pound filo dough
½ pound butter, melted and clarified
1 pound Monterey Jack cheese
½ pint large curd cottage cheese
4 ounces cream cheese
2 eggs

Open filo dough and cut in half. Put half of the melted butter in a 9″ x 13″ casserole dish. Put half of the filo into dish and tuck in to lay flat. Mix together the cheeses and eggs and gently spread on the filo. Place remaining half of filo on top of cheese mixture and tuck in to keep flat. Pour remaining half of the butter on top, sealing edges. Bake in 350 degree oven for 30-45 minutes until golden brown. Let stand 10 minutes before cutting. Great for brunches or luncheons.

Easy Souffle

8 servings.

½ cup butter or margarine
5 eggs
¼ cup flour
½ teaspoon baking powder
2 7 ounce cans Ortega diced chiles
8 ounces low fat cottage cheese
½ pound Monterey Jack cheese, shredded
Salsa

Melt butter. Beat eggs and then add to butter. Slowly sift flour and baking powder into above mixture. Add remaining ingredients, and combine. Grease a 9″ x 13″ pan. Pour in mixture and bake for 30 minutes in a 400 degree oven. When done, the top should be golden. Serve with favorite salsa on top.

Bunch of Brunch Casserole

8 to 10 servings.

1 bell pepper, chopped
1 onion, chopped
½ pound mushrooms, sliced
1 tablespoon margarine
1 package frozen creamed spinach
1 dozen eggs, whipped
½ pound grated Swiss cheese
½ pound grated Monterey Jack cheese
1 pound bacon, cooked, crumbled
Salt and pepper to taste
¼ teaspoon paprika

Saute pepper, onion and mushrooms in margarine. Add creamed spinach. In a frying pan, cook eggs until almost done. Add vegetable mixture and half of the cheese and half of the bacon. Add salt, pepper and paprika. Mix. Pour into a 9″ x 13″ pan. Top with remaining bacon and cheese. Bake in 375 degree oven until cheese melts.

May be prepared one day ahead, refrigerated and then baked.

Breakfast Potato Pie

6 servings.

6 eggs
¼ cup grated onion
½ teaspoon thyme
¼ teaspoon salt
¼ teaspoon pepper
3 cups frozen hash brown potatoes
1 cup shredded Swiss or
cheddar cheese
½ cup chopped ham or bacon bits
½ cup chopped green pepper
1 tomato, chopped or thinly sliced

Heat oven to 350 degrees. Grease a 9″ pie pan. In a bowl, combine eggs, onion, thyme, salt and pepper. Beat well. Stir in potatoes, cheese, ham and green pepper. Pour into pie pan. Bake for 45 minutes or until set. Garnish with tomatoes.

Bountiful Brunch

12 servings.

12 slices white bread, crusts removed
Margarine, softened
2-3 tablespoons butter or
½ cup butter or margarine
½ pound fresh mushrooms, trimmed and sliced
2 cups thinly sliced yellow onions
1½ pounds mild Italian sausage
¾-1 pound cheddar cheese, grated
5 eggs
2½ cups milk
3 teaspoons Dijon mustard
2 teaspoons brown mustard
1 teaspoon ground nutmeg
1 teaspoon salt
⅛ teaspoon pepper
2 tablespoons finely chopped fresh parsley

Spread the bread with the softened butter and set aside. In a 10"-12" skillet, melt ½ cup butter. Add and brown the mushrooms and onions and saute over medium heat for 5-8 minutes or until tender. Set aside. Cook the sausage and cut into bite-sized pieces.

In a greased 9" x 13" casserole, layer half of the bread, mushroom mixture, sausage, and cheese. Repeat the layers, ending with the cheese. In a medium-sized mixing bowl mix the eggs, milk, both mustards, nutmeg, salt and pepper. Pour over the sausage and cheese casserole. Cover the casserole and refrigerate overnight.

When ready to bake, sprinkle the parsley evenly over the top of the casserole and bake, uncovered, in a preheated 350 degree oven for 1 hour or until bubbly. Serve immediately with a fruit salad and crusty bread.

Deviled Egg Casserole

10 to 12 servings.

12 hard boiled eggs
⅓ cup mayonnaise
½ teaspoon curry powder
½ teaspoon paprika
½ teaspoon salt
¼ teaspoon dry mustard

Cut eggs in half lengthwise and scoop out yolks. Combine egg yolks with mayonnaise and spices. Use a small spoon or pastry tube to put the filling back in the whites. Arrange in casserole baking dish.

Sauce:
2 tablespoons butter
2 tablespoons flour
1 10.75 ounce can cream of mushroom soup
10.5 ounces milk
¼ pound small shrimp or crab
¾ cup shredded sharp cheddar cheese
Bread crumbs

Sauce:
Over low heat, make sauce of butter, flour, soup, milk, shrimp and ½ cup of cheese. Pour over eggs in casserole. Cover casserole with bread crumbs and remaining cheese. Bake at 350 degrees for 30-45 minutes.

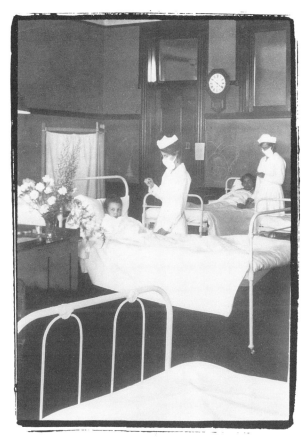

General patient ward, early 1900's

soups and salads

Turtle Soup From Beans

Soak over night one quart of black beans; next day boil them in the proper quantity of water, say a gallon, then dip the beans out of the pot and strain them through a colander.

Then return the flour of the beans, thus pressed, into the pot in which they were boiled.

Tie up in a thin cloth some thyme, a teaspoonful of summer savory and parsley, and let it boil in the mixture. Add a tablespoonful of cold butter, salt and pepper. Have ready four hard-boiled yolks of eggs quartered, and a few force meat balls; add this to the soup with a sliced lemon, and half a glass of wine before serving the soup.

This approaches so near in flavor to the real turtle soup that few are able to distinguish the difference.

The White House Cookbook © 1887

Two Melon Soup

7 cups.

1 ripe cantaloupe, peeled,
seeded and coarsely chopped
2 tablespoons lemon juice, or to taste
½ honeydew melon, peeled,
seeded and coarsely chopped
3 tablespoons lime juice, or to taste
1½ teaspoons minced mint leaves,
Sour cream (optional)
Mint sprigs

In food processor or blender, combine cantaloupe and lemon juice and process in batches until smooth. Chill in covered bowl at least 3 hours or overnight.

In food processor or blender, combine honeydew melon, lime juice and mint leaves and process in batches until smooth. Chill in covered bowl at least 3 hours or overnight. Do not combine melon mixtures.

Using two measuring cups containing each melon soup, pour equal amounts of soups at same time into individual chilled bowls. Garnish with sour cream and sprig of mint.

§ *Calories: 82 Fat: 1.4gm Cholesterol: 8mg Sodium: 21mg*

Cold Chili Soup

4 servings.

1-2 tablespoons minced onion
¼ cup sherry
1 teaspoon prepared horseradish
½ teaspoon chili powder
1 10.5 ounce can tomato soup
1 cup cold water
½ pint sour cream
½ cup finely minced green pepper

Combine all ingredients, except for the green pepper, in the blender and whirl until smooth. Chill 3-4 hours before serving. Garnish with minced green pepper. Can be served with avocado spread on French bread.

Pumpkin Soup

4 servings.

2 tablespoons butter
4 scallions, chopped
1 small onion, sliced
1½ pounds fresh pumpkin, peeled and diced
4 cups chicken stock
½ teaspoon salt
2 tablespoons flour
1 tablespoon butter
¾ cup light cream
1 tablespoon butter
Toasted croutons

Melt 2 tablespoons butter in a large saucepan, add scallions and onion. Cook them gently until they are almost soft but not brown. Add pumpkin, chicken stock and salt. Simmer the pumpkin until it is soft. Stir in 2 tablespoons flour kneaded with 1 tablespoon butter and bring the soup to a boil. Rub the soup through a fine sieve or puree it in a blender. Correct the seasoning, and add ¾ cup hot light cream and 1 tablespoon butter. Heat the soup just to the boiling point and serve it garnished with tiny toasted croutons.

Broccoli Soup

4 to 6 servings.

1 small onion, chopped
2 tablespoons butter or margarine
1 14.5 ounce can double strength chicken broth
3 cups chopped broccoli, fresh or frozen
1 cup half and half (milk may be substituted)
2 tablespoons flour
Dash of curry powder
Salt and pepper to taste
¼ cup sour cream (optional)

In a medium saucepan, saute onion in butter until soft. Add chicken broth and broccoli and simmer until broccoli is tender. Pour mixture into blender or food processor. Process until pureed. Add half and half, flour and curry powder. Blend until smooth. Return to pan and reheat until just simmering. Add salt and pepper to taste. Serve with a dollop of sour cream, if desired.

Diana's Carrot Soup

6 cups.

2 tablespoons margarine
1 medium onion, diced
2½ cups chicken broth
1 pound carrots, peeled and sliced
1¾ cups diced potatoes
1½ cups milk
Salt and pepper to taste

Melt margarine in large saucepan. Add onion, saute 5 minutes. Add broth, carrots and potatoes. Simmer until tender. Puree in blender. Return to pan. Add milk. Season to taste and warm.

§ *Calories: 163 Fat: 7.4gm Cholesterol: 8mg Sodium: 621mg*

Mushroom Soup Supreme

6 servings.

½ pound fresh mushrooms, sliced
¼ cup butter
2 cups chicken stock
3 egg yolks
1 cup half and half or light cream
¼ teaspoon salt
⅛ teaspoon pepper
2 tablespoons sherry

Set aside 6 mushroom slices for garnish. Saute remaining mushrooms in butter for 5 minutes. Pour stock, mushrooms and egg yolks in blender. Cover and run on high speed for 2 seconds. Pour into saucepan. Add cream, salt and pepper. Stir over low heat until hot and slightly thickened. Add sherry.

Pour into individual soup bowls and serve immediately. Garnish each cup with mushroom slice.

Seafood Bisque

6 servings.

4 tablespoons butter
Small onion, finely chopped
½ cup chopped celery
2 tablespoons chopped parsley
1 teaspoon dry mustard
2 bay leaves
½ teaspoon paprika
½ teaspoon oregano
½ teaspoon tarragon
1 teaspoon thyme
1 teaspoon basil
½ cup flour
2 cups clam nectar
½ cup white wine
1 cup chili sauce
1 cup tomato puree
1½ cups sour cream
2 cups half and half
½ lemon with rind
Dash of tabasco
Dash of Worcestershire sauce
4 ounces clams
6 ounces baby shrimp
2 ounces scallops
8 ounces white fish
(sole, perch, cod, etc.)
2 ounces crabmeat

Melt the butter and saute the onion, celery, parsley, and next 7 spices. Set aside. Make a roux of the flour, clam nectar, and white wine. Cook down briefly, and then combine the roux and sauteed ingredients. Add the next 7 ingredients. Stir to blend. Add remaining seafood, and heat briefly to cook all seafood.

Zucchini-Italian Sausage Soup

2 quarts.

¾ pound mild Italian sausage,
casings removed
1½ teaspoons olive oil
1 medium onion, diced
1 green pepper, diced
1 stalk celery, diced
2 cups diced tomatoes
2 cups canned tomato sauce
1 quart beef stock
½ cup burgundy wine
1 teaspoon Worcestershire sauce
1 teaspoon garlic powder
1 teaspoon basil
1 teaspoon oregano
1 teaspoon black pepper
1 teaspoon onion powder
½ teaspoon seasoned salt
1 tablespoon beef or chicken base
3 medium-sized zucchini, sliced
½ cup grated romano cheese

Saute sausage in oil. Add onion, pepper, celery, and saute until tender. Add tomatoes, tomato sauce, stock and wine and bring to a boil. Reduce heat and simmer for 30 minutes. Add remaining ingredients except cheese and simmer for a bit longer. Serve with romano cheese.

Potato Leek Soup

4 servings.

2 large potatoes,
peeled and finely diced
2 large leeks, thinly sliced
4 cups chicken broth
½ teaspoon salt
¼ teaspoon fresh ground black pepper
4 small round loaves of bread, unsliced
2 cloves garlic, crushed
4 teaspoons olive oil
4 tablespoons grated parmesan cheese
¼ cup heavy whipping cream
⅛ teaspoon grated nutmeg
Chopped parsley

In a large pot combine potatoes, leeks, chicken broth, salt and pepper. Over high heat, heat to boiling. Reduce heat to low, cover and simmer for 15 minutes. Meanwhile, make bread bowls by taking a small sharp knife and cut into loaf, leaving ¾″ edge. Hollow out the center and reserve leftover bread for croutons. Rub inside with garlic; brush with olive oil and sprinkle with cheese.

Place hollowed-out loaves and bread "lids" on a cookie sheet and bake in 350 degree oven for 15 minutes or until cheese melts.

When the soup has simmered, use a sieve to strain soup into another pan. Place solids in blender or food processor with knife blade and process until smooth; return to soup in pan. Stir in heavy cream and nutmeg; heat through.

Spoon hot soup into bread bowls and top with chopped parsley.

§ *Calories: 356 Fat: 8.6gm Cholesterol: 45mg Sodium: 820mg*

Winter Vegetable Chowder

6 cup servings.

1　cup chopped onion
½　cup sliced celery
2　tablespoons butter
1　large potato,
peeled and cut in ½″ cubes
1　cup sliced carrots
2　cups water
1　beef bouillon cube
1　teaspoon salt
½　teaspoon crushed basil
¼　teaspoon black pepper
1½　cups sliced zucchini
1　7 ounce can whole kernel corn,
undrained
1　tablespoon flour
⅔　cup evaporated milk
½　cup shredded cheddar cheese

In a Dutch oven, saute onion and celery in butter, just until tender. Add potatoes, carrots, water, bouillon, salt, basil and pepper. Heat to boiling. Reduce heat, cover and boil gently for 30 minutes. Stir in zucchini and corn with liquid. Boil gently for 30 minutes.

Combine flour with small amount of evaporated milk. Stir until smooth. Blend in remaining milk and add to vegetables. Cook, stirring constantly over medium heat until mixture just comes to a boil. Remove from heat and add cheese. Stir until melted.

Ladle into serving bowls and sprinkle with additional cheese if desired.

§　*Calories: 192 Fat: 8gm Cholesterol: 20mg Sodium: 631mg*

Crab Bisque

8 to 10 servings.

1　6 ounce can crab meat
½　pound flaked imitation crab or
fresh equivalent
1½　cups dry sherry
3　10.5 ounce cans tomato soup
2　15 ounce cans split pea soup
2　cups milk

Soak crab in sherry for at least 1 hour. Combine remaining ingredients, add crab mixture. Bring to a boil, stirring occasionally. Serve.

California Chili

10 servings.

½ pound pinto beans
5 cups canned tomatoes
1 pound green peppers, chopped
¼ cup butter or margarine
1¼ pounds chopped onions
2-3 cloves garlic, crushed
½ cup chopped parsley
2 tablespoons salt
2½ pounds coarsely ground beef
1 pound ground lean pork
⅓ cup chili powder
1½ teaspoons pepper
1½ teaspoons cumin seed or powder

Wash beans, bring to a boil in 6 cups water. Boil for 2 minutes, then let stand for 1 hour. Simmer covered in same water until tender, about 45 minutes. Add tomatoes and simmer 5 minutes. Saute green peppers in butter for 5 minutes. Add onion, cook until tender and yellow, stirring often. Add garlic and parsley.

Cover bottom of large skillet with salt and saute meat until brown. Drain off fat. Add meat to onion mixture; stir in chili powder and cook 10 minutes. Add this to beans and add remaining spices. Simmer covered for 1 hour. Cook uncovered 30 minutes.

Acapulco Vegetarian Soup

4 servings.

2 medium tomatoes, cut into 1″ cubes
1 large russet potato, cut into 1″ cubes
1-3 fresh serrano or jalapeno chiles (according to taste), seeded and very thinly sliced
1 large carrot, thinly sliced
1 medium onion, thinly sliced
Juice of ½ lemon
1 small bunch fresh cilantro
Salt and pepper

Place all ingredients, including salt and pepper to taste, in a large soup pot or stew kettle. Add 1 quart water, bring to a boil and simmer, covered, for 30 minutes or until potatoes are tender. Adjust seasoning.

§ *Calories: 68 Fat: .3gm Cholesterol: 0mg Sodium: 166mg*

Hearty Harvest Soup

6 to 8 servings.

½ pound ground turkey
½ pound mild Italian sausages, casings discarded
½ cup chopped onion
6 cups regular strength beef broth
1 cup tomato juice
1 cup dry red wine
3 large firm-ripe tomatoes, cored and chopped
3 large carrots, peeled and sliced
2 cups coarsely chopped zucchini
1 tablespoon Worcestershire sauce
2 teaspoons dry oregano leaves
1 teaspoon liquid hot pepper seasoning

In a 3-4 quart pan over medium-high heat, combine turkey, sausage, and onion. Stir often until meat is lightly browned, about 15 minutes. Transfer meat mixture with a slotted spoon to drain on paper towels. Discard fat in pan; wipe pan clean. Return meat mixture to pan; add broth, tomato juice, wine, tomatoes, carrots, zucchini, Worcestershire sauce and oregano. Cover and simmer over medium heat until the carrots are tender to bite, 20-30 minutes. Add liquid hot pepper seasoning to taste.

Hot Tomato Bouillon

6 to 8 servings.

2 10.5 ounce cans tomato soup
2 10.5 ounce cans beef bouillon
4½ cups tomato juice
2 teaspoons sugar
2 teaspoons Worcestershire sauce
1 teaspoon dehydrated onion flakes (optional)
1 tablespoon dry sherry (optional)

Combine all ingredients in saucepan and heat to boiling. May add dehydrated onion flakes or sherry if desired.

§ *Calories: 94 Fat: .9gm Cholesterol: 9mg Sodium: 1223mg*

Cream Mongole Soup

4 to 6 servings.

1 10.75 ounce can condensed
tomato soup
1 10.75 ounce can condensed
pea soup
¾ cup water
1 cup milk
2 teaspoons Worcestershire sauce
5 tablespoons sherry

Combine soups and water. Heat over low heat, stirring until mixture is smooth. Add milk slowly and stir in Worcestershire sauce. Add sherry. Heat thoroughly.

Rice-Shrimp Gumbo

6 servings.

¾ cup chopped onion
¾ cup chopped green pepper
¼ cup water
1 28 ounce can tomatoes,
drained and diced
½ teaspoon bottled minced garlic, or
⅛ teaspoon garlic powder
Several dashes of hot pepper sauce
¼ teaspoon paprika
⅛ teaspoon pepper
1½ cups water
1 6.25 ounce packaged quick-cooking
long grain and wild rice mix
1 16 ounce package frozen shrimp

In a large saucepan, combine onion, green pepper and ¼ cup water. Bring to a boil and simmer, covered for 3-5 minutes. Add tomatoes to onion mixture along with spices. Stir in 1½ cups water and both packets from rice mix. Bring mixture to a boil. Add frozen shrimp. Return to boil. Reduce heat. Cover and simmer 5 minutes. Serve with additional hot pepper sauce.

§   *Calories: 243 Fat: 2.2gm Cholesterol: 131mg Sodium: 418mg*

Dieters Meal-In-One Vegetable Soup

8 to 10 servings.

1 tablespoon poly-unsaturated oil
3 cloves garlic, minced
1 stalk celery, chopped
1 bell pepper, seeded and
chopped coarsely
2 unscraped carrots,
sliced into rounds
3 unpeeled red potatoes, sliced thin
1 cup yellow squash, chopped coarsely
2 zucchini cut into rounds
2 leaves chard or spinach
2 cups fresh tomatoes or 1 pound can
stewed tomatoes and juice
2 quarts chicken broth
2 tablespoons fresh parsley
1 tablespoon diced celery and leaves
1 teaspoon oregano
1 teaspoon basil
½ teaspoon cayenne
Tabasco to taste
1 cup cooked rice or pasta
Parmesan cheese

Over the lowest heat in a 6 quart pot, place oil and vegetables in the order given. As you add the vegetables turn up the heat. Stir. Cook a few minutes. Now add the liquids and seasonings. Keep the heat high until you have a full rolling boil. Lower heat and boil gently, uncovered, for 20 minutes. Add rice or pasta, cook for an additional 10 minutes. Cover and let stand until ready to eat. Serve with a dusting of parmesan cheese.

§ *Calories: 171 Fat: 6.2gm Cholesterol: 1mg Sodium: 161mg*

Potato, Ham & Cheese Soup

4 to 6 servings.

2-3 medium russet potatoes, peeled and sliced thick
2-3 stalks celery, cut in ½″ pieces
2-3 carrots, peeled and cut in ¼″ pieces
1 medium onion, chopped
1 cup cooked ham, cut in bite-size pieces
1 tablespoon fresh parsley
2-3 tablespoons butter
¼-½ cup milk
1-1½ cups grated cheddar cheese
Salt and pepper

Place potatoes, celery, carrots, onions, ham, parsley and 1 tablespoon butter in large saucepan. Add water to 1″ below all ingredients. Bring to boil and stir; reduce heat to simmer and cover with lid. Cook approximately 15-20 minutes until vegetables are tender. Do not overcook. Add just enough milk to change broth to white color. Stir in cheese and additional butter, if desired. Heat to melt cheese. Serve immediately. Best when served the same day as made.

Ellie's Manhattan Clam Chowder

4 servings.

2 tablespoons oil
3 ribs celery, diced
1 carrot, diced
½ cups chopped fresh or canned tomatoes
2 cups diced potatoes
2 cups water
1-2 cans minced clams, drained
Salt, pepper and thyme to taste

Lightly saute in oil the celery, onion and carrot. Add tomatoes, potatoes and water. Simmer 30 minutes. Add clams, bring to a boil and remove from heat. Let rest 2 minutes before adding salt, pepper and thyme to taste.

Zucchini Cheese Chowder

8 servings.

½ pound zucchini, sliced
2 onions, sliced
1 15 ounce can garbanzo beans, drained
1 16 ounce can chopped tomatoes, undrained
¼ cup butter or margarine
1⅓ cups dry white wine
2 teaspoons minced garlic
1 teaspoon minced basil leaves
1 bay leaf
Salt and pepper to taste
1 cup shredded Monterey Jack cheese
1 cup grated parmesan cheese
1 cup whipping cream or milk

Combine zucchini, onions, beans, tomatoes, butter, wine, garlic, basil and bay leaf in a 3 quart baking dish. Cover and bake in 400 degree oven for 1 hour, stirring once halfway through. Season to taste with salt and pepper. Stir in cheeses and cream. Bake 10 minutes longer.

Portuguese Kale Soup

6 to 8 servings.

1 cup black eyed peas
¼ pound salt pork
1 large onion, chopped
2 pounds kale, cut in pieces
2 packages Linguisa (Portuguese sausage), sliced
2 cups cubed potatoes
1 clove garlic

Rinse beans. Boil beans, salt and onion until almost tender. Add kale, Linguisa, potatoes and garlic. Cook until potatoes are tender.

Green Soup

8 to 10 servings.

2 10 ounce packages frozen peas
2 10 ounce packages frozen
       chopped spinach
1 onion, chopped
1 bay leaf
2 tablespoons chopped parsley
4 cups chicken broth
2 cups milk or half and half
1 teaspoon curry powder
1 tablespoon soy sauce

Cook vegetables, bay leaf and parsley in one-fourth of the broth for 20-25 minutes. Remove bay leaf and then puree vegetables in food processor. Add remaining broth, milk and seasonings. Pour mixture into saucepan and bring to a simmer. Do not boil.

§ *Calories: 144 Fat: 4gm Cholesterol: 8mg Sodium: 776mg*

Hungarian Sauerkraut Soup

4 to 6 servings.

1 29 ounce can sauerkraut
1 28 ounce can peeled tomatoes
½ cup barley
1 apple, peeled and sliced
2 pounds chuck or soup meat,
       diced into 1″ pieces
2 cloves garlic, diced
6 bay leaves
Sour salt to taste (citric acid—
available at gourmet food stores)
4 cups water

Put all ingredients in large pot and cook for several hours. Add more water if soup becomes too thick. Season to taste.

Pasta Salad

8 to 10 servings.

1 16 ounce package pasta
1 cup sugar
1 cup white vinegar
1 cup oil
1 teaspoon celery seed
1½ cups diced green onions
1 cup shredded carrots
1 cup finely sliced green peppers
1 cup thinly sliced radishes
1 cup thinly shredded cauliflower
1-2 cups cooked, cubed chicken
(optional)

Bring water to boil and cook pasta according to package directions and drain.

Combine sugar, vinegar, oil and celery seed in saucepan and bring to boil. Add to drained pasta and refrigerate for 12 hours. Add vegetables and refrigerate for an additional 6-12 hours. Chicken may be added if desired.

Sumi Salad

6 to 8 servings.

¼ cup sugar
1 teaspoon black pepper
1 teaspoon salt
1 cup oil
8 tablespoons rice vinegar
2 tablespoons oil
1¼ cups sliced or slivered almonds
¼ cup sesame seeds
8 green onions, finely sliced
1 head cabbage, finely chopped
2-2½ 3 ounce packages ramen,
uncooked

Make dressing by combining sugar, pepper, salt, oil and vinegar. Mix well. Set aside.

Heat oil in skillet and toast almonds and seeds until lightly browned. Combine with onions, cabbage, noodles and dressing. Cover and chill several hours for flavors to blend.

Elegant Fresh Vegetable Salad

4 servings.

½ pound fresh French green beans, washed and trimmed and cut into ½" pieces
1¼ cups cooked corn kernels
1 cup cherry tomatoes, chopped and drained
⅔ cups diced, cooked artichoke bottoms
4 large lettuce leaves
Tomato slices

Dressing:
2 tablespoons white wine vinegar
2 tablespoons fresh lemon juice
½ teaspoon seasoned salt
¼ teaspoon white pepper
1-2 tablespoons whipping cream
¼ cup vegetable oil
¼ cup olive oil
3-4 tablespoons minced fresh basil leaves

Steam beans until tender but still crunchy. Drain and cool. In a large bowl combine green beans, corn, chopped tomatoes and artichoke pieces with about ¼ cup dressing (or to taste).

To serve, arrange one lettuce leaf on each of four plates; mound vegetables in center of each and surround attractively with half slices of tomato.

Dressing:
In a small mixing bowl, combine vinegar, lemon juice, salt, pepper and whipping cream. Add oils in a slow stream, whisking until well blended. Stir in 3-4 tablespoons minced fresh basil leaves. Refrigerate dressing at least 3 hours before using.

Sonoma Chicken Salad

6 servings.

6 cups Boston and Bibb lettuce,
cleaned and cut
1 cup trimmed watercress
1 head Belgian endive
2 tomatoes, chopped
1 bunch green onions, chopped
4 slices bacon, cooked and crumbled
2 cups cooked, cubed chicken, cooled
1 avocado, cubed
2 garlic cloves, peeled
¼ cup chopped scallion
¼ cup chopped fresh dill
4 ounces mild goat cheese
½ cup mayonnaise
½ cup milk
¼ teaspoon thyme
½ teaspoon salt
Dash pepper
Dash tabasco

Combine the lettuce, watercress, endive, tomatoes, green onions, bacon, chicken and avocado in a large salad bowl. In a food processor, combine the remainder of the ingredients and process until smooth. Toss with salad ingredients and serve immediately.

Apple Cabbage Slaw

6 to 8 servings.

1 head cabbage
2 red or green apples
1 cup mayonnaise
¼ cup sugar or
2 packages artificial sweetener
2 cups mini-marshmallows (optional)

Shred the cabbage. Core and dice apples, leaving the skin on. Toss with mayonnaise and sugar. Add mini-marshmallows if desired and toss again.

Red, Red Salad

10 to 12 servings.

2 3 ounce packages raspberry jello
2 cups boiling water
1 16 ounce can jellied cranberry sauce
2 tablespoons lemon juice
1 12 ounce package frozen raspberries
Whipped cream

Dissolve jello in boiling water. Add cranberry sauce in "chunks." Let stand 5 minutes and beat with mixer until dissolved. Mixture tends to splatter.

Stir in lemon juice, add raspberries, including any juice, and beat once more. Put in mold and chill until firm. Serve with whipped cream in center.

Artichoke Rice Salad

6 servings.

1 7 ounce package of any chicken rice mix
1 6 ounce jar marinated artichoke hearts, cut in half
4 green onions, sliced, including tops
½ green or red pepper, diced
12 green stuffed (pimento) olives, sliced
1 8 ounce can water chestnuts, cut in halves or quarters
½ cup mayonnaise
½ teaspoon curry powder

Cook rice according to package directions, omitting butter. Let cool. Drain the artichokes, reserve marinade. In a large bowl, place onions, peppers, olives, artichokes and water chestnuts. Add cooked rice.

Blend the artichoke marinade, mayonnaise and curry powder and combine with rice mixture. Refrigerate at least 4 hours. Best if refrigerated overnight.

Pasadena Spinach Salad

6 servings.

1½ ounces of liquid pasteurized eggs (available in the freezer section of most grocery stores)
1 tablespoon parmesan cheese
½ teaspoon salt
Dash white pepper
2 teaspoons Dijon-type mustard
3 tablespoons lemon juice
1 teaspoon Worcestershire sauce
1 teaspoon sugar
¼ cup oil
2 bunches spinach
2 eggs, hard cooked and finely chopped
6 slices bacon, cooked crisp and crumbled

Beat together pasteurized eggs, cheese, salt, pepper, mustard, lemon juice, Worcestershire sauce and sugar. Blend well. Add oil and beat thoroughly. (If not used immediately, cover and refrigerate.)

Wash spinach thoroughly, breaking off leaves from stems. Dry leaves well. Place in a salad bowl. Sprinkle with egg and bacon. Add dressing and toss lightly, but thoroughly.

Bing Cherry Salad Mold

16 to 18 servings

3 16 ounce cans bing cherries
3 3 ounce black cherry jello
2½ cups hot water
2½ cups dry sherry
2¼ cups cherry syrup, from bing cherries
1½ cups sour cream
1½ cups sliced almonds

Drain cherries, save 2¼ cups syrup. Dissolve jello in hot water. Add sherry and cherry syrup until thickened. Add cherries, sour cream and almonds. Pour into a large mold and chill until firm. Unmold on a bed of lettuce.

Salad Nicoise

4 servings.

2 small white rose potatoes, cooked and diced
½ 10 ounce package frozen cut green beans, cooked
2 hard boiled eggs, quartered
1 head Boston lettuce
6 red-leaf lettuce leaves
2 tomatoes, cut in eighths
1 3 ounce can pitted medium black olives
6 slices red onion, separated into rings
1 tablespoon capers
1 6.5 ounce can solid white tuna
⅔ cup olive oil
⅓ cup red wine vinegar or lemon juice
¼ teaspoon dry mustard
2-3 teaspoons Dijon mustard
½ teaspoon basil
½ teaspoon sugar
⅛ teaspoon salt
⅛ teaspoon pepper
1 clove garlic, crushed

Cook potatoes, beans and eggs ahead of time. Chill lettuce, tomatoes, olives, onions, capers and tuna until ready to assemble. To make dressing place olive oil, vinegar, mustards, basil, sugar, salt, pepper and garlic in a large jar and shake to combine.

When ready to serve, place all ingredients in an extra-large salad bowl and toss with dressing to combine.

Grape & Carrot Slaw

6 servings.

2 cups shredded carrots
1½ cups halved grapes, seeded if necessary
½ cup thinly sliced celery
¼ cup chopped green pepper
¼ cup mayonnaise
¼ cup sour cream
2 teaspoons prepared horseradish
1 teaspoon honey
½ teaspoon lemon juice
¼ teaspoon salt

Combine carrots, grapes, celery and green pepper. Make dressing by combining remaining ingredients. Add dressing to slaw; mix well. Cover and refrigerate at least 1 hour before serving.

24 Hour Frozen Salad

12 servings.

2 21 ounce cans white seeded cherries, drained
2 cups pineapple chunks, drained
2 8 ounce cans mandarin oranges, drained
2 cups marshmallows, cut fine
2 eggs, beaten
4 tablespoons lemon juice
4 tablespoons sugar
2 tablespoons butter
1 cup whipping cream

Mix fruits and marshmallows.

Put eggs in double boiler and add lemon juice and sugar. Cook, stirring constantly until thick and smooth. Remove from stove. Add butter. Cool in pan of water.

Whip cream until stiff peaks form. When dressing is cold, fold in whipped cream and fruit. Freeze for 24 hours.

Los Angeles Cole-Slaw

10 to 12 servings.

1 head cabbage
¾ cup mayonnaise
3 tablespoons sugar
1½ tablespoons white wine vinegar
⅓ cup oil
⅛ teaspoon garlic powder
⅛ teaspoon onion powder
⅛ teaspoon dry mustard
⅛ teaspoon celery seed
Dash black pepper
1 tablespoon lemon juice
½ cup half and half
¼ teaspoon salt

Shred cabbage. Mix remaining ingredients together and pour over cabbage. Chill for 6 hours or overnight.

Salmon Vegetable Salad

6 servings.

1 7.5 ounce can salmon, drained and flaked
1 cup canned peas
½ cup grated carrots
¼ cup chopped celery
¼ cup chopped sweet pickles
6 ripe olives, chopped
1 tablespoon lemon juice
1 tablespoon French dressing
¼ cup mayonnaise
6 large lettuce leaves
6 sprigs of parsley

Combine salmon, peas, carrots, celery, pickles and olives. Blend lemon juice, French dressing and mayonnaise together. Pour dressing on vegetables and toss. Serve on lettuce leaves. Garnish with parsley if desired.

§ *Calories: 210 Fat: 12.8gm Cholesterol: 7mg Sodium: 514mg*

Easy Caesar Salad

8 servings.

½ cup olive oil
1 clove garlic, crushed
2 eggs, raw or
3 ounces liquid pasteurized eggs
3 tablespoons lemon juice
1 tablespoon Worcestershire sauce
½ teaspoon salt
¼ teaspoon pepper
3 tablespoons anchovy paste
2 cups bread cubes
¼ cup olive oil
2 heads Romaine lettuce,
washed and chilled
¼ cup crumbled blue cheese
¼ cup grated parmesan cheese

Combine ½ cup olive oil, garlic, pasteurized eggs, lemon juice, Worcestershire sauce, salt, pepper and anchovy paste in jar and refrigerate. Saute bread cubes in ¼ cup olive oil until crisp. Drain on paper towels and set aside. Tear lettuce into large salad bowl. Add blue cheese, parmesan and croutons. Shake dressing and pour over salad. Toss and serve immediately.

Raisin Broccoli Salad

6 servings.

1½ pounds fresh broccoli, chopped
4 ounces red onion, sliced thin
3 ounces raisins
3 ounces sunflower seeds
8 ounces mayonnaise
2 tablespoons sugar
2 tablespoons lemon juice
8 slices bacon, cooked and crumbled

Combine broccoli, onions, raisins and sunflower seeds. Combine mayonnaise, sugar and lemon juice. Fold dressing into salad mixture. Add bacon before serving.

Charlie's Tuna Salad

12 servings.

2 10 ounce packages petite frozen peas,
thawed and drained
2 13.5 ounce cans tuna,
water packed, drained
3 cups chopped celery
1 9.5 ounce jar cocktail onions,
cut in half, drained
1 cup sour cream
1 cup mayonnaise
1½ tablespoons soy sauce
2 tablespoons lemon juice
¼ teaspoon garlic salt
2 cups chow mein noodles
Toasted almonds

Combine all ingredients except for the chow mein noodles and almonds. Before serving, add noodles and toss salad. Garnish with toasted almonds.

Green Pea Salad

10 servings.

1 20 ounce package petite green peas,
thawed and drained
1 cup chopped celery
2 green onions, including tops,
chopped
1½ pints sour cream
½ cup soybean bacon bits
1 cup salted peanuts

Mix the peas, celery, onions and sour cream. Let stand overnight in refrigerator. Just before serving, fold in the bacon bits and salted peanuts.

Quick Fix Ham Salad

6 servings.

3 tablespoons grated fresh horseradish
or 5 tablespoons prepared horseradish
1 tablespoon white vinegar
2 cups water
6 small red-skinned potatoes, washed and cubed
1 pound piece baked Virginia ham, cubed
3 ribs celery, sliced
2 medium carrots, sliced
2 scallions, sliced
½ cups mayonnaise
2 tablespoons chopped parsley

If using fresh horseradish, soak in vinegar 15 minutes. Meanwhile, in 1 quart saucepan, over high heat, bring water to a boil. Add potatoes; reduce heat to low and simmer until fork-tender, about 15 minutes. In large bowl, combine ham, celery, carrots and scallions. Drain potatoes; add to bowl. In medium bowl, stir together horseradish mixture, mayonnaise and parsley. Pour dressing over salad; toss to coat.

Rice Salad

6 to 8 servings.

1 package Chicken Rice-A-Roni
2 small jars marinated artichoke hearts
⅓ teaspoon curry powder
4 scallions, chopped
Diced green pepper to taste

Prepare Rice-A-Roni as directed on package. Cool. Add remaining ingredients. Lightly toss salad to combine. Make one day ahead and chill.

§ *Calories: 137 Fat: .9gm Cholesterol: 0mg Sodium: 458mg*

Quick Fruit Salad

6 to 8 servings.

1 head butter lettuce
2 nectarines, peeled and sliced
1 cup blueberries
1 cup cantaloupe, cubes or balls

Dressing:
⅓ cup olive oil
3 tablespoons raspberry vinegar
3 tablespoons fresh orange juice
(about one orange)
¼ teaspoon salt
⅛ teaspoon cracked pepper

Tear the lettuce into pieces and place in a large bowl. Add fresh fruit and toss.

Dressing:
Mix dressing ingredients and refrigerate. Toss the salad lightly with the vinaigrette and serve immediately.

§ *Calories: 120 Fat: 9.3gm Cholesterol: 0mg Sodium: 78mg*

Tangy Golden Apple Salad

4 to 6 servings.

2 cups ¾″ cubed
Golden Delicious apples
2 zucchini, cut into ½″ slices
2 carrots, cut into ¼″ slices,
cooked crisp-tender
¼ cup chopped green onion
2 tablespoons chopped parsley
¼ cup white vinegar
2 tablespoons oil
½ teaspoon crushed basil leaves
¼ teaspoon salt
Pepper to taste

Combine apples, zucchini, carrots, onion and parsley; mix well. Chill thoroughly. Mix vinegar, oil, basil, salt and pepper and add to vegetables. Allow to marinate for at least 1 hour before serving.

§ *Calories: 51 Fat: 2.9gm Cholesterol: 0mg Sodium: 65mg*

Spinach / Sprouts & Fruit Salad

6 servings.

3 bunches spinach, washed and stem free
2 baskets strawberries, washed and hulled
2 cups bean sprouts, washed
4 navel oranges, peeled and segmented
1 cup Honey Dressing (or to taste)

Honey Dressing:
⅔ cup sugar
1 teaspoon dry mustard
1 teaspoon paprika
¼ teaspoon salt
1 teaspoon celery seed
⅓ cup honey
5 tablespoons vinegar
1 tablespoon lemon juice
1 tablespoon green onion
1 cup salad oil

Toss the spinach, strawberries, bean sprouts and oranges in large bowl with Honey Dressing. Garnish with a few of the sprouts, strawberries and orange segments if desired.

Honey Dressing:
Make dressing in a food processor fitted with a steel blade. Mix all ingredients for dressing except for oil, then add oil slowly through tube. Makes 2 cups and can be kept for some time in refrigerator.

Chicken Salad with
Mandarin Oranges & Pecans

6 servings.

½ cup coarsely chopped pecans
2 cups cooked chicken, sliced
1 bunch watercress,
tough stems removed
1 11 ounce can mandarin oranges,
chilled and drained
2 scallions, sliced
6 tablespoons olive oil
2 tablespoons raspberry or
red wine vinegar
½ teaspoon salt
¼ teaspoon freshly ground pepper

Preheat oven to 325 degrees. Spread out pecans on a small baking sheet. Bake to 10-15 minutes, until lightly toasted.

In a small bowl, combine chicken, watercress, oranges, scallions and toasted pecans. Drizzle oil, vinegar, salt and pepper onto salad. Toss to coat.

Peanut Broccoli Salad

6 to 8 servings.

8 tablespoons mayonnaise
2 tablespoons Italian salad dressing
4 cups washed and diced raw broccoli
8 tablespoons pickle relish
8 tablespoons diced onion
2 eggs, hard boiled and chopped
Salt and pepper
1 cup chopped peanuts

In a bowl, thin mayonnaise with salad dressing. Add remaining ingredients except peanuts. Toss to coat with dressing. Add salt and pepper to taste. Add peanuts just before serving.

Zesty Waldorf Turkey Salad

6 to 8 servings.

2 cups shredded light and dark turkey meat, about ½" x 2"
2 large celery ribs cut in matchstick pieces, ¼" x 1"
1 large Granny Smith or other tart apple, diced in ¼" pieces
1 cup large walnut pieces
½ cup golden raisins
1½ cups nonfat plain yogurt
1 tablespoon finely grated orange zest
2 teaspoons dried tarragon
Salt and pepper

In a large bowl, combine turkey, celery, apple, walnuts and raisins. In a smaller bowl, combine yogurt, orange zest, tarragon, salt and pepper. Mix well and toss over turkey salad. Adjust seasonings to taste. Cover; refrigerate at least 1 hour before serving.

Krab Salad

4 servings.

1 pound imitation crab, flaked
1 stalk celery, diced
10 water chestnuts, diced
2 tablespoons sliced olives
2 tablespoons drained capers
3-4 dashes Worcestershire sauce
1 tablespoon fresh lemon juice
2 tablespoons mayonnaise
Lemon-herb seasoning to taste

Combine all ingredients. Mix carefully until well blended and serve.

§ *Calories: 190 Fat: 7.3gm Cholesterol: 27mg Sodium: 1383mg*

Cucumber & Shrimp Sunomono

8 servings.

4 large cucumbers
2 teaspoons salt
4 ounces Saifun (bean threads)
¾ cup sugar or
12 packages of sugar substitute
2 cups rice vinegar
Slivered sweet ginger
Small shrimp

Peel and slice cucumbers in half lengthwise. Remove seeds and slice paper thin. Add salt and let stand. Soak Saifun in hot water for 20 minutes. Drain and rinse thoroughly in cold water. Cut in 2″ lengths. Squeeze excess moisture out of cucumbers and combine in large bowl with Saifun. Sprinkle sugar over cucumbers and add vinegar. Add sweet ginger and small shrimp as desired.

§ *Calories 105 Fat: .3gm Cholesterol: 15mg Sodium: 607mg*

Broccoli Salad

6 servings.

1 bunch broccoli (2 pounds),
washed and cut in small bite-size pieces
⅓ cup shredded cheddar cheese
1 small red onion, minced
10-12 slices of bacon,
cooked and crumbled
½ cup mayonnaise
¼ cup sugar
1 tablespoon red wine vinegar

Mix broccoli, cheese, onion and bacon. Place mayonnaise, sugar and red wine vinegar in a blender or food processor fitted with a steel blade and blend well.

Pour dressing over salad and toss. Marinate for at least 2 hours.

Hot Chicken Salad

6 servings.

3 chicken breasts,
cooked and shredded
1 10.5 ounce can cream of
chicken soup, undiluted
¾ cup mayonnaise
1 cup diced celery
2 cans sliced water chestnuts, drained
3 eggs, hard boiled
½ cup slivered almonds
½ teaspoon salt
Onion to taste
⅓ cup sherry
⅓ cup sliced mushrooms
Crushed potato chips

Combine all ingredients except for potato chips. Place mixture in a casserole dish. Spread potato chips over top. Bake in 375 degree oven for 30 minutes.

Baked Pineapple Chicken Salad

10 servings.

3 cups cooked and cubed chicken
1⅓ cups chopped celery
⅓ cup French dressing
2½ cups shredded cheddar cheese
1 13.5 ounce can pineapple tidbits,
drained
½ cup slivered toasted almonds
¾ cup sour cream
¾ cup mayonnaise
1½ teaspoons prepared mustard
½ teaspoon salt
1 cup crushed potato chips

Marinate chicken and celery in dressing for 1 hour, drain if necessary. In large bowl, combine chicken, celery, 1½ cups cheese, pineapple and almonds.

Blend sour cream, mayonnaise, mustard and salt. Pour over chicken mixture, blending gently. Spoon salad into 7″ x 10″ baking dish. Combine potato chips and remaining cup of cheese. Use to cover top of salad. Bake in 325 degree oven for 30-40 minutes until hot.

Andre's Hot Brie Dressing

2 to 3 cups.

10 ounces Brie cheese
½ cup olive oil
2 shallots, minced
2 cloves garlic, minced
½ cup sherry wine vinegar
2 tablespoons lemon juice
4 teaspoons Dijon mustard
Freshly ground pepper

Cut Brie into small pieces and bring to room temperature. In large heavy skillet, warm oil over heat for 10 minutes. Add shallots and garlic and cook just until translucent, about 5 minutes. Do not brown. Stir in vinegar, lemon juice and mustard. Add cheese and stir until smooth. Season with pepper. Serve hot, over mixed greens.

Cheddar Dressing

2 cups.

1 cup shredded cheddar cheese
1 tablespoon prepared horseradish
¼ cup apple juice or apple cider
1 cup sour cream

In small bowl with whisk, combine all ingredients. Chill until ready to serve. Use on tossed green salad. May also be used on winter fruit such as pear or apple slices.

Fruit Dip Dressing

1 cup.

½ cup sour cream
¼ cup orange marmalade
½ cup finely chopped walnuts

Combine all ingredients together. Serve with fresh fruit slices.

Carinne's Fruit Salad Dressing

1½ pints.

1½ cups sugar
2 teaspoons dry mustard
3 tablespoons onion juice
⅔ cup vinegar
2 cups salad oil (not olive oil)
3 teaspoons poppy seeds

Mix dry ingredients. Add onion juice and vinegar and process in a blender. Drip oil slowly into blender. Stir in poppy seeds and store in refrigerator. Serve on fresh fruits.

Fruit Salad Dressing

½ cup.

8 ounces nonfat plain yogurt
3 tablespoons honey (or to taste)
Dash of cinnamon

Mix ingredients together and use over seasonal fruit. In the winter, use coconut and toasted pecans with apples, pears, oranges and bananas. In the summer, use over melons, berries and grapes.

§ *Calories: 40 Fat: 0mg Cholesterol: 1mg Sodium: 22mg*

1-2-3 Fruit Dressing

2 cups.

1 egg, well beaten
1 cup sugar
Juice and grated rind of 1 lemon
Juice and grated rind of 1 lime
Juice and grated rind of 1 large orange

Combine all ingredients in a saucepan. Cook over medium heat, stirring constantly, until boiling. Boil 1 minute. Remove and cool. Store in a covered jar in the refrigerator.

Refreshing Citrus-Mint Dressing

1½ cups.

⅓ cup orange juice
1 tablespoon sugar
2 teaspoons cornstarch
Salt to taste
1 egg, slightly beaten
½ teaspoon grated orange peel
2 tablespoons lemon juice
⅓ cup sour cream
1 teaspoon finely chopped fresh mint, or
½ teaspoon dried

Combine orange juice, sugar, cornstarch and salt in saucepan. Heat just to boiling, stirring constantly. Remove from heat and cool slightly. Whisk in egg, orange peel and lemon juice. Fold in sour cream and mint. Cover and refrigerate until ready to use.

Blue Ribbon French Dressing

2 cups.

1 teaspoon seasoned salt
1 teaspoon sugar
1 teaspoon paprika
½ teaspoon pepper
½ cup red wine vinegar
1½ cups olive oil
2 teaspoons chopped parsley
¼ teaspoon chopped oregano

Combine all ingredients in jar. Shake well and refrigerate. Keeps well in refrigerator.

Creamy French Dressing

1½ cups.

1 cup mayonnaise
½ cup catsup
2 tablespoons cider vinegar

Mix all ingredients. Stir until smooth. Cover and chill.

Creamy Italian Dressing

1½ cups.

1 cup mayonnaise
¼ cup milk
2 tablespoons red wine vinegar
1 clove garlic, minced
½ teaspoon dried oregano

Mix all ingredients. Stir until smooth. Cover and chill.

Creamy Mexican Dressing

2 cups.

1 cup mayonnaise
1 cup prepared chunky salsa

Mix all ingredients. Stir until smooth. Cover and chill.

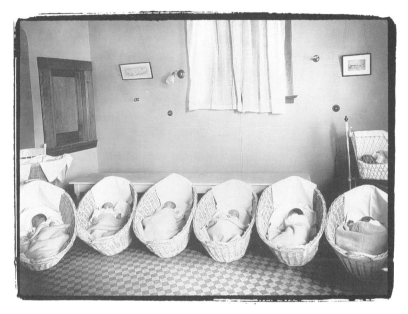

Newborn nursery, 1914 - 1915

seafood

Boston Fry

Prepare the oysters in egg batter and fine cracker meal; fry in butter over a slow

fire for about ten minutes; cover the hollow of a hot platter with tomato sauce;

place the oysters in it, but not covering; garnished with chopped

parsley sprinkled over the oysters.

The White House Cookbook © 1887

Grilled Trout
with Beer & Caper Sauce

6 servings.

3 tablespoons butter
3 tablespoons flour
¾ cup hot water
¾ cup hot beer
½ teaspoon salt
½ cup capers
1 tablespoon chopped parsley
Juice of 1 lime
6 1 pound pieces rainbow or
brook trout

In saucepan, melt butter and stir in flour. Gradually whisk in hot water and the beer, whisking until sauce is smooth. Add salt, capers, parsley and lime juice and keep warm.

Split fish and grill until flaky, about 10-12 minutes. Serve hot with sauce.

Piquant Fish Fillets

4 servings.

⅓ cup orange juice
2 tablespoons malt vinegar
1 tablespoon soy sauce
4 fish fillets (sole, flounder or
orange roughy)
1 cup chopped broccoli
1 cup sliced carrots
1 celery stalk, cut into 1″ pieces
4 orange slices

In small bowl, mix orange juice, vinegar and soy sauce. Set aside. Place each fillet in the center of a separate 12″ square of foil. Arrange vegetables on each fillet. Pour sauce over each. Fold foil over each fillet, securing seams tightly. Place on cookie sheet. Bake in 450 degree oven for 30 minutes.

With a spatula, transfer individual servings to heated plates, open packets, spoon a small amount of sauce over each. Garnish with orange slices.

§ *Calories: 175 Fat: 1.9gm Cholesterol: 77mg Sodium: 353mg*

Halibut with Orange Sauce

4 servings.

2 9 ounce halibut steaks (1″ thick)
2 teaspoons vegetable oil
1 teaspoon salt-free extra-spicy
   herb seasoning blend
   Orange slices

Orange Sauce:
1 teaspoon grated orange rind
¼ cup orange juice
½ teaspoon curry powder
¼ teaspoon ground cumin
1 cup low fat yogurt
2 tablespoons catsup

Brush fish evenly on each side with oil and sprinkle with seasoning mix, place on broiler rack. Fish should be 4″ from heat. Broil 5-7 minutes on each side, or until fish flakes evenly with fork.

Place fish on serving platter; spoon sauce over and garnish with orange slices.

Orange Sauce:
In small saucepan, over medium high heat, cook orange rind and juice, curry and cumin, 3 minutes. Remove from heat, cool slightly. Add yogurt and catsup; cook gently over low heat, stirring occasionally, until heated through.

Company Fish

4 servings.

3 tablespoons melted butter
1 onion, thinly sliced
1½ pounds red snapper fillets
½ cup mayonnaise
¼ cup grated parmesan cheese
2 tablespoons lemon juice
1 teaspoon Worcestershire sauce
½ teaspoon paprika
½ teaspoon salt
   Oregano
   Chopped parsley

Pour butter into bottom of 9″ x 13″ baking dish. Arrange onion evenly over bottom of dish. Place fish in single layer over onion. Combine mayonnaise, cheese, lemon juice, Worcestershire sauce, paprika and salt. Spread evenly over top of fish. Sprinkle with oregano and parsley. Bake in 350 degree oven for approximately 35-40 minutes or until fish flakes easily with fork.

Tangerine Fillet of Sole

4 servings.

8 tablespoons butter or margarine
2 teaspoons tangerine peel, grated
½ cup tangerine juice
1 teaspoon lemon juice
1 tablespoon finely chopped parsley
1 tablespoon finely chopped chives
½ bay leaf, crumbled
1 tangerine, peeled, sectioned and seeded
⅛ teaspoon salt
⅛ teaspoon pepper
¼ cup flour
1 pound fish fillets
4 parsley sprigs

Combine 5 tablespoons of the butter, tangerine peel and juice, lemon juice, chopped parsley, chives and bay leaf in saucepan. Simmer over low heat until slightly thickened, about 2 minutes. Add tangerine sections.

Salt, pepper and flour fish fillets. Fry in 3 tablespoons hot butter in a skillet until browned on both sides and fish flakes easily. Serve on hot platter with tangerines and sauce. Garnish with parsley.

Fillet of Sole Parisienne

8 servings.

½ cup butter
½ cup white wine vinegar
1 tablespoon Dijon mustard
2 teaspoons salt
2 teaspoons lemon juice
1 teaspoon savory
½ teaspoon pepper
1 clove garlic, crushed
1-2 drops tabasco sauce
8 fillets of sole
Salt to taste
Pepper to taste

In small saucepan, combine all ingredients, except fillets, salt and pepper. Simmer over low heat for 5 minutes. Place fillets in shallow baking dish. Season with salt and pepper. Pour sauce on top and broil until fillets flake with a fork, about 10 minutes.

Orange Roughy with Sesame

4 servings.

1 large egg white
⅓ cup sesame seeds
4 orange roughy fillets,
skinned and boned
2 tablespoons salad oil
Lemon wedges
Soy sauce

Put egg white in a shallow 9″ or 10″ wide pan and beat with a fork until slightly frothy. Put sesame seeds in another shallow 9″ or 10″ wide pan. Rinse fish and pat dry. Dip fillets on 1 side only in egg white, lift out, and let drain briefly. Then lay egg-moistened side in sesame seeds, coating heavily and equally. Lay fillets, seeds up, side by side on sheet of wax paper.

Place a 10″ x 15″ rimmed baking pan in 500 degree oven and heat for about 5 minutes. Swirl oil in pan; then lay fish, seeds down, in pan. Bake on lowest oven rack, uncovered, until fish flakes readily when prodded with a fork in thickest part and seeds on bottom are lightly browned, about 8 minutes. Transfer fillets, seed side up, onto 4 dinner plates. Serve with lemon wedges and soy sauce to add to taste.

§ *Calories: 219 Fat: 13.9gm Cholesterol: 23mg Sodium: 426mg*

Low-Calorie Halibut Marengo

4 servings.

1½ pounds halibut steaks
½ teaspoon salt
1 tomato, diced
½ cup tomato juice
¼ cup water
1 tablespoon lemon juice
¼ cup sliced mushrooms
¼ cup diced celery
1 tablespoon minced onion
¼ teaspoon thyme
Dash black pepper
1 tablespoon chopped parsley

Sprinkle halibut with salt and place in shallow baking dish. Spoon tomato over halibut. Combine tomato juice, water, lemon juice, mushrooms, celery, onion, thyme and pepper. Bring to boil and simmer 5 minutes. Pour hot mixture over halibut. Cover and bake at 375 degrees for 15-20 minutes, or until halibut flakes easily. Garnish with chopped parsley.

§ *Calories: 203 Fat: 4gm Cholesterol: 54mg Sodium: 484mg*

Sarah's Salmon Diable

6 servings.

6 large 1″ thick salmon steaks
⅓ cup butter, softened
2 tablespoons lemon juice
2 teaspoons Dijon mustard
⅛ teaspoon cayenne pepper
1 tablespoon minced parsley
Olive oil
Liquid Smoke

Soak salmon in 1 quart salted water for 30 minutes. While salmon is soaking, beat butter until creamy. Gradually beat in lemon juice until mixture is fluffy. Beat in mustard, cayenne pepper and parsley. Set aside.

Brush salmon with olive oil and liquid smoke. Grill 6″ above hot coals. Turn once with a wide spatula. Cook until fillets flake in center, about 10 minutes. Top each fillet with an equal portion of butter mixture.

Salmon Timbales

5 servings.

1 7.5 ounce can salmon
Half and half, slightly warmed
4 eggs, beaten
¼ teaspoon salt
⅛ teaspoon pepper
¾ cup shredded cheddar cheese
¼ cup finely minced onion
2 tablespoons chopped parsley

Drain salmon, reserving liquid; remove bones; flake meat. Add half and half to reserved salmon liquid to equal 1¼ cups. Combine with eggs, salt and pepper. Stir in salmon and remaining ingredients. Pour into 5 (6 ounce each) custard cups. Place in pan of hot water with water level to the top of the egg mixture. Bake in 325 degree oven for 35-45 minutes or until knife inserted near center comes out clean. Let stand 10 minutes before unmolding onto serving plates.

Nippy Salmon in Baskets

6 servings.

1 8.75 ounce can corn kernels, drained
4 cups lightly packed shredded romaine lettuce
2½-3 cups cooked salmon, broken into large pieces
(about 1½ pounds of salmon steaks, with bones and skin removed)
6 tortilla baskets
(available at most bakeries and Mexican specialty stores)

Chile Mayonnaise:
1½ cups mayonnaise
1 4 ounce can diced green chiles
Cayenne pepper to taste

In a bowl, lightly mix corn, romaine, and salmon; spoon into hot tortilla baskets. Add Chile Mayonnaise over salmon in baskets to taste.

Chile Mayonnaise:
In a food processor or blender, whirl mayonnaise and green chiles until smooth. Stir in cayenne to taste. If made ahead, cover and refrigerate for up to 1 day. Makes 1¾ cups.

Salmon Steaks with Spinach

4 servings.

4 salmon steaks, 1″ thick
Salt and pepper
1 teaspoon dill weed
4 tablespoons butter
1 large onion, chopped
1 clove garlic, minced or mashed
2 pounds fresh spinach, cut into 1″ strips
Lemon wedges

Arrange salmon on a lightly greased pan. Broil 4″ from heat for 5 minutes. Turn steaks and season with salt and pepper; sprinkle with dill weed and dot with about 1 tablespoon butter. Broil steaks for about 5 minutes more or until fish flakes when prodded with a fork.

Meanwhile, in large frying pan, saute the onion and garlic in the remaining butter until limp. Stir in the spinach with water that clings to the leaves. Cover pan and cook over high heat for about 3 minutes; stir occasionally.

To serve, arrange spinach on platter or individual plates and lay salmon steaks and lemon wedge on top.

Shrimp Brew

4 servings.

1 pound cleaned fresh or frozen shelled and deveined medium shrimp
1 bay leaf
6 sprigs dill or 1 teaspoon dill weed
1 garlic clove, minced
Juice of ½ lemon
¼ teaspoon whole peppercorns
⅛ teaspoon dried red pepper flakes
1 cup beer
Melted butter

Combine all ingredients in a saucepan. Over high heat, bring to a full rolling boil. Cover; remove from heat. Let stand 4 minutes or until shrimp are pink and curled. Drain. Serve hot with melted butter if desired.

§ *Calories: 141 Fat: 1.3gm Cholesterol: 221mg Sodium: 259mg*

Stir-Fry
Sesame Shrimp & Asparagus

6 servings.

1½ pounds asparagus
1 tablespoon sesame seeds
⅓ cup oil
2 small onions, sliced
1½ pounds shrimp, peeled and cleaned
4 teaspoons soy sauce
Salt to taste

Trim asparagus and cut into 2″ pieces. Set aside. In large skillet or wok, toast sesame seeds over medium heat until golden, stirring and shaking occasionally. Remove seeds and set aside.

Add oil to skillet. Over medium heat, stir-fry asparagus, onions and shrimp until shrimp turn pink and vegetables are tender yet crisp, about 5 minutes. Stir in seeds and soy sauce. Salt to taste.

§ *Calories: 271 Fat: 15.1gm Cholesterol: 172mg Sodium: 404mg*

Shrimp with Garden Fresh
Vegetables & Fruit

4 to 6 servings.

1 pound snow peas, trimmed and stringed
6 tablespoons sweet butter
2 large, firm, tart apples, peeled and cut into thick slices
2 tablespoons granulated sugar
½ cup finely minced yellow onion
2 pounds medium-size raw shrimp, shelled and deveined
¾ cup dry white wine or vermouth
⅔ cup prepared Dijon-style mustard
¾ cup heavy cream or creme fraiche

Bring a large pot of salted water to a boil and drop in the cleaned snow peas. When tender but still crunchy, after about 3 minutes, drain them and plunge immediately into ice water. This will stop the cooking process and set their bright green color. Reserve.

In a large skillet melt 2 tablespoons of the butter and saute the apple slices over medium heat until tender but not mushy, about 5 minutes. Sprinkle slices with the sugar and raise the heat, rapidly turning apple slices until they are brown and lightly caramelized. Using a spatula, remove slices from the skillet and reserve. In the same skillet melt remaining 4 tablespoons butter and gently cook the minced onion, covered, over medium heat until tender and lightly colored, about 25 minutes. Raise the heat, add the shrimp, and stir and toss them rapidly in the butter until they are firm and pink, about 3 minutes. Do not overcook. Remove shrimp from the skillet and reserve.

Pour the wine or vermouth into the skillet and over high heat reduce it by two thirds. Turn down the heat and stir in the mustard with a wire whisk. Pour in the cream or creme fraiche and simmer uncovered, stirring occasionally, for 15 minutes or until sauce is reduced slightly.

Drain snow peas thoroughly and pat dry with paper towels. Add them, along with reserved apples and shrimp, to the mustard-cream sauce and simmer together for 1 minute. Serve immediately.

Shrimp Chippewa

7 servings.

56 medium-size raw shrimp, peeled
4 cloves garlic, chopped
1½ cups sliced fresh mushrooms
1½ cups butter
¼ cup chopped parsley
1¼ cups chopped green onions
7 cups chicken stock
French bread

Saute shrimp, garlic and mushrooms with ½ cup butter. Add parsley and green onions to the chicken stock. Combine with shrimp and mushroom mixture and bring to a boil. Take off heat, add remaining butter while stirring constantly. The butter will thicken the sauce.

Serve in soup plates with French bread for dipping.

Shrimp Stuffed Sole

6 servings.

⅓ cup cocktail shrimp
1 egg beaten
½ cup seasoned bread crumbs
¼ cup diced celery
Salt and pepper to taste
6 pieces sole or white fish

Sauce:
3 tablespoons margarine
3 tablespoons flour
Dash salt
1½ cups milk
⅓ cup dry white wine
1 cup grated Swiss or
Monterey Jack cheese
Chopped parsley

Combine cocktail shrimp, egg, bread crumbs, celery, salt and pepper to make stuffing. Spoon about ¼ cup of stuffing onto each fish fillet. Roll up and place in glass baking dish, seam side down. Cover dish with wax paper. Cook in microwave on high for 8-10 minutes or until fish flakes easily. Drain off any liquid that accumulates.

Sauce:
Place margarine in glass measure and microwave 30 seconds. Stir in flour, salt, milk and wine until smooth. Heat uncovered for 3 minutes or until thickened. Stir in cheese and blend until smooth. Spoon over fish and sprinkle with parsley to garnish.

Shrimp & Crabmeat Jambalaya

10 servings.

¾ teaspoon salt
¾ teaspoon ground cayenne pepper
½ teaspoon black pepper
1 pound peeled small shrimp
4 tablespoons unsalted butter
1 8 ounce can tomato sauce
2 cups finely chopped green onions, tops and bottoms
½ cup finely chopped green pepper
¼ cup finely chopped parsley
2 tablespoons minced garlic
2 bay leaves
¼ teaspoon dried thyme leaves
2 cups clam juice
1 cup uncooked converted rice
1 teaspoon ground hot vinegar peppers (optional)
1 teaspoon salt
½ teaspoon black pepper
½ pound crabmeat (imitation can be used)

Combine ¾ teaspoon salt, ground cayenne pepper and black pepper in a small bowl. Place shrimp in a medium-size bowl. Add the blended seasonings. Mix and work it in with your hands. Cover and refrigerate until ready to use.

Melt butter in large Dutch oven over high heat. Stir in tomato sauce and cook until tomato is noticeably darker and butter separates out of mixture, making large puddles of red oil, about 8 minutes. Stir so mixture doesn't scorch. Stir in green onions, bell peppers, parsley, garlic, bay leaves and thyme; cook 2 minutes stirring constantly. Stir in the clam juice and rice. Cook about 2 minutes more, stirring once or twice. Stir in vinegar peppers if desired. Add salt and black pepper. Bring to a boil, then reduce heat to simmer slowly. Cover pan and cook about 15 minutes without stirring. Add shrimp and crabmeat, stirring and scraping pan bottom well. Re-cover pan and remove from heat. Let sit covered about 10 minutes. Stir well, remove bay leaves.

Savvy Shrimp Scampi Over Pasta

4 servings.

½ pound dry angel hair pasta
1¾ cups defatted chicken broth
2 tablespoons chopped garlic
4 tablespoons chopped shallots
4 tablespoons chopped parsley
1 pound peeled and deveined shrimp,
tail shells left on
Freshly ground black pepper to taste

Bring a large pot of water to a boil for the pasta. Add pasta to boiling water. Cook according to directions.

Combine broth, garlic and 3 tablespoons each of shallots and parsley in a large saucepan. Bring slowly to a simmer; cook 2 minutes. Add shrimp to broth, stir well and cook for 2½-3½ minutes, or until shrimp are cooked through. Add remaining shallots.

Drain pasta; divide evenly among large shallow plates. Arrange shrimp over pasta and spoon broth sauce over shrimp. Sprinkle with pepper; garnish with remaining parsley.

§ *Calories: 360 Fat: 4.4gm Cholesterol: 172mg Sodium: 616mg*

Clam Linguini

4 to 6 servings.

2 tablespoons olive oil
3 medium onions, coarsely chopped
3 cloves garlic, minced
2 10 ounce cans baby clams
½ cup dry white wine
Freshly ground pepper to taste
3 tablespoons lemon juice
9 ounces angel hair pasta,
cooked and drained

Heat oil in skillet and saute onions and garlic for about 10 minutes until onions have softened. Add the juice from clams, then wine and bring to a boil. Continue boiling to reduce liquid by half, about 20 minutes. Add clams, pepper and lemon juice and cook just enough to heat thoroughly. Serve clam sauce over pasta.

New England Sherry Scallops

8 servings.

1½ pounds sea scallops
½ cup butter or margarine
2 tablespoons sherry
¼ teaspoon salt
¼ teaspoon white pepper
½ cup crushed cracker crumbs
1 tablespoon chopped parsley

Lightly grease scallop shells or individual baking dishes. Do not rinse scallops. Divide scallops evenly among shells. Melt butter and pour all but 2 tablespoons over scallops. Sprinkle with sherry, salt and pepper.

Bake in 350 degree oven for 20 minutes. Remove from oven. Mix cracker crumbs with remaining melted butter. Top scallops with buttered crumbs and parsley. Place under broiler for 1 minute to heat.

Deviled Crab-Avocado

6 servings.

½ cup slivered almonds
2 tablespoons butter
2 tablespoons flour
½ teaspoon salt
1 cup milk
2 teaspoons prepared mustard
1 teaspoon Worcestershire sauce
2 tablespoons lemon juice
2 cups cooked crab
(can use imitation crab)
3-4 avocados

Toast almonds for 10 minutes in 300 degree oven. Melt butter in small saucepan. Add flour and salt. Blend in milk and cook over medium heat until sauce thickens. Add mustard, Worcestershire sauce, lemon juice, crab and half of the almonds. Reheat but do not boil.

Peel avocados and cut in half lengthwise. Slice each half into 5 or 6 slices lengthwise and arrange in fan on small plate. Spoon crab over avocado. Sprinkle with remaining toasted almonds and serve immediately.

Deviled Crab Cakes

6 servings.

3 tablespoons butter or margarine
4½ tablespoons flour
½ teaspoon salt
¼ teaspoon pepper
¾ cup light cream
1 egg yolk
½ teaspoon A-1 sauce
2 tablespoons chopped parsley
6 ounces crab meat
½ cup fine bread crumbs
2 eggs, beaten
½ cup coarse bread crumbs
1 tablespoon butter

Melt butter in small saucepan; add flour, salt and pepper. Mix. Pour in cream and cook until very thick, stirring constantly. Remove from heat. Add egg yolk and A-1 sauce; mix well. Add parsley and crab meat. Blend well.

Chill mixture 3 hours. Form into 6 balls or patties and dip each one into fine bread crumbs. Coat with beaten eggs and then dip into coarse bread crumbs. Let stand at room temperature for 1 hour. Saute patties in butter until golden brown. Serve with tartar sauce and lemon wedges.

Easy Paella

4 to 6 servings.

1 cup hot water
3 tablespoons olive oil
1 package Lipton's Spanish rice and sauce mix
1 ripe tomato, chopped
2 zucchini, sliced ¼" thick
1½ cups sea scallops
1 10 ounce can whole baby clams with juice
4 ounces imitation crab
1 cup bay shrimp
3-4 dashes hot pepper sauce

In large saucepan, combine hot water, olive oil, rice and sauce mix. Bring to boil. Add the tomatoes, zucchini, sea scallops, clams with juice, crab, bay shrimp, and hot pepper sauce. Cover and simmer until rice is tender, approximately 45 minutes.

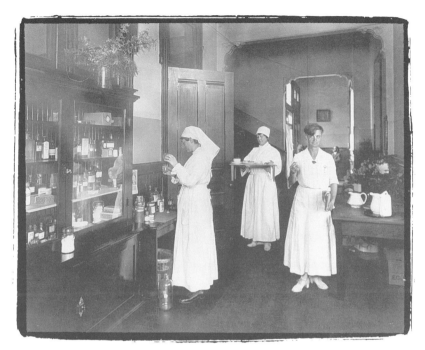

"Pharmacy," early 1900's

poultry

Chicken Poly Pie

One quart of flour, two teaspoonfuls of cream of tartar mixed with the flour, one

teaspoonful of soda dissolved in a teacupful of milk; a teaspoonful of salt; do not use

shortening of any kind, but roll out the mixture half an inch thick, and lay on it minced

chicken, veal or mutton. The meat must be seasoned with pepper and salt and be free

from gristle. Roll the crust over and over, and put it on a buttered plate

and place in a steamer for half an hour. Serve for breakfast or lunch,

giving a slice to each person with gravy served with it.

The White House Cookbook © 1887

Sherry Mustard Chicken or Turkey

4 servings.

4 small chicken breasts, skinless,
boneless or 4 slices of turkey breast
1 tablespoon olive oil
2 heaping tablespoons Dijon mustard
1 cup very dry sherry
2 tablespoons fresh lemon juice
1 teaspoon ground sage
1 tablespoon onion powder
White pepper to taste
¼ cup chopped chives
½ cup low sodium chicken broth

Pound chicken breasts between 2 sheets of wax paper. Breasts should be thin to cook quickly. In large skillet, saute chicken in olive oil until thoroughly cooked. Do not overcook. Remove breasts from pan and place in a glass dish. Cover and keep warm.

To skillet, add mustard, sherry, lemon juice, sage, onion powder and pepper. Bring to a boil stirring well to blend ingredients; add chives, then chicken broth. Return breasts, with accumulated juices, back to pan and cook until thoroughly heated. Can be made 1 hour ahead and gently reheated.

§ *Calories: 260 Fat: 7gm Cholesterol: 73mg Sodium: 294mg*

Easy Chicken Cacciatore

4 to 6 servings.

1 6 ounce can tomato paste
1 package Lawry's spaghetti sauce mix
(extra thick)
4 pounds chicken thighs
(approximately 12)

Prepare spaghetti sauce according to directions on package, but eliminate butter or oil. Place chicken thighs in bottom of 9″ x 13″ baking dish. Pour cooked sauce over chicken and bake in 350 degree oven, stirring occasionally for 1 hour. Serve over cooked noodles.

Chinese Chicken Pita

14 servings.

2 pounds chicken cut in thin strips
2 tablespoons vegetable oil
2 cups broccoli cut into 1″ pieces
2 cups sliced onions
2 cups sliced green peppers
4 tablespoons soy sauce
4 tablespoons dry sherry
2 teaspoons cornstarch
1 teaspoon sugar
1 cup bean sprouts
2 cups shredded iceberg lettuce
14 6″ round pita breads

In a large skillet or wok, saute chicken strips in hot oil along with broccoli, onions and green peppers.

Combine soy sauce, dry sherry, cornstarch and sugar to make sauce mixture. When chicken is thoroughly cooked, add sauce mixture and mix well.

Wash and drain bean sprouts and thinly slice lettuce. Put a small amount of each in a pita bread and fill with some of the chicken mixture.

§ *Calories: 286 Fat: 5.7gm Cholesterol: 48mg Sodium: 283mg*

Chicken Sweet & Tangy

4 servings.

½ cup butter
¼ cup Worcestershire sauce
1 large clove garlic, minced
½ cup red currant jelly
1 tablespoon Dijon mustard
1 cup orange juice
1 teaspoon powdered ginger
3 dashes tabasco
1 chicken, quartered

In saucepan, combine butter, Worcestershire sauce, minced garlic, currant jelly, Dijon mustard, orange juice, powdered ginger and tabasco. Heat, stirring until jelly is melted and sauce is smooth. Cool.

Put chicken in a baking dish. Pour sauce over and let marinate for 2-3 hours. Preheat oven to 350 degrees. Cover chicken and cook in the oven for 1 hour. Uncover, increase oven temperature to 400 degrees and baste frequently until chicken is an even dark brown. Serve with pilaf if desired.

Aunt Sadie's Chicken Pot Pie

6 servings.

½ onion, diced
⅓ cup butter
⅓ cup flour
½ teaspoon salt
1½ cups half and half
1½ cups chicken broth
4 cups cooked cubed chicken
1 cup frozen peas
1 cup diced carrots, cooked
1 package biscuits (can make your own baking powder biscuits)

Cook onion in butter. Blend in flour and salt. Stirring constantly, add half and half and then the broth. Cook until smooth and thickened. Add chicken, peas and carrots and heat to bubbling. Add seasonings as desired. Pour into 2½ quart casserole. Top with biscuits. Bake in 450 degree oven for 10-15 minutes, or until filling is bubbly and biscuits are completely cooked.

Microwave Onion-Orange Chicken

4 servings.

6 ounce can orange juice concentrate, thawed
1 envelope dry onion soup mix
½ cup dry bread crumbs
3 pounds cut-up chicken pieces

In a pie plate, place orange juice concentrate. Combine onion soup mix and dry bread crumbs in a plastic bag; mix together. Using 3 pounds of cut-up chicken pieces, dip each piece in orange juice, then shake in the bag of crumb mixture to coat well.

Place chicken in microwaveable 12″ x 8″ baking dish. Sprinkle remaining crumbs on top of chicken; cover with paper towel. Microwave on high 15-20 minutes, or until chicken is fork tender and juices run clear. Rearrange chicken once during cooking.

Herbed Bar-B-Que Chicken

4 servings.

4 chicken breast halves
¼ teaspoon summer savory or
¾ teaspoon fresh
1 teaspoon thyme or
1 tablespoon fresh
½ teaspoon sage or
1½ teaspoons minced fresh
½ teaspoon rosemary or
1½ teaspoons minced fresh
¼ teaspoon marjoram or
¾ teaspoon fresh
3 tablespoons minced fresh parsley
1 teaspoon grated lemon rind
⅛ teaspoon red cayenne pepper
⅓ cup olive oil
Salt and pepper to taste
1 lemon, cut into wedges

Skin, bone and flatten chicken breasts to ¼" thickness. Combine all herbs, spices, lemon rind and oil. Rub cutlets with mixture. Arrange in shallow dish. Cover and chill overnight.

Sprinkle cutlets with salt and pepper to taste. Grill on well oiled rack over glowing coals for 2-3 minutes on each side. Garnish with lemon wedges.

Benny's Jalapeño Chicken

6 to 8 servings.

1 10.75 ounce cream of chicken soup
1 pint sour cream
1 8 ounce package cream cheese
1 cup jalapeño peppers (from a jar)
2½ cups chopped chives
8 chicken breasts, skinned and boned

Combine all ingredients except for the chicken breasts. Place chicken breasts in baking pan and pour sauce over the chicken. Bake in 325 degree oven for 1 hour 15 minutes. Serve over rice.

Exotic Ginger Chicken Breasts

4 to 6 servings.

3 whole chicken breasts, skinned,
boned and split
¼ cup all-purpose flour
6 tablespoons butter
2 green onions, finely chopped
½ teaspoon minced fresh ginger
3 tablespoons chutney
⅓ cup Madeira
¾ cup chicken broth
¾ cup whipping cream
2 tablespoons chopped
crystallized ginger

Rinse chicken and pat dry. Pound each breast half between plastic with a flat mallet until ¼″ thick. Dust chicken pieces lightly with flour; shake off excess.

In a 10″-12″ frying pan, melt 3 tablespoons of the butter over medium-high heat. Add chicken, a portion at a time. Cook, turning, until browned on both sides, 4-6 minutes. Transfer chicken, as cooked to a warm platter. Add more butter to pan as needed.

To pan, add onions, fresh ginger, chutney, Madeira and broth. Boil over high heat, stirring, until reduced by half, about 5 minutes. Add cream and boil, stirring, until reduced to about 1¼ cups. Pour sauce over chicken and sprinkle with crystallized ginger.

Chicken Rebecca

2 to 4 servings.

4 tablespoons butter
2 chicken breasts, skinned,
boned and cut in half
1 cup dried apricots
4 tablespoons orange marmalade

Place butter into a shallow baking dish. Place chicken on top. Arrange apricots around chicken and spread 1 tablespoon of marmalade on top of each piece of chicken. Cover pan with foil. Bake in 350 degree oven for 45 minutes or until tender.

Chicken Royale Cutlets

4 servings.

4 chicken breast halves
1 cup finely chopped pecans
2 ounces romano cheese, grated
½ cup dried bread crumbs
1 teaspoon sage
Pepper to taste
1 egg
2 tablespoons water
2 tablespoons butter
1 tablespoon oil

Skin, bone and flatten chicken to ¼″ thickness. On a dinner plate combine nuts, cheese, bread crumbs, sage and pepper. In small bowl, beat egg and water. Coat each cutlet with nut mixture, then dip in egg, then nut mixture again. In large skillet, heat butter and oil together. Saute each cutlet just until done, about 2-3 minutes on each side.

Herbed Chicken

6 servings.

1 cup chopped fresh mint, dill and parsley in equal proportions
2 cloves minced garlic
6 chicken breasts, skinned, boned and halved (about 4½ pounds)
Salt and freshly ground black pepper
2 lemons
4 tablespoons sweet butter

Mix herbs and garlic together in a small bowl. Flatten chicken breasts by pressing them gently against the work surface with the palm of your hand. Place each breast on a piece of foil and season with salt and pepper. Sprinkle herb and garlic mixture over chicken breasts. Slice lemons and arrange 2 or 3 slices over each breast. Dot with butter and seal the packets. Set on a baking sheet. Set packets in the middle of the oven and bake at 350 degrees or 30 minutes. Serve in packets.

Boursin Stuffed Chicken

2 to 4 servings.

**2 whole medium chicken breasts,
skinned and boned**

Stuffing:
**1 5 ounce package boursin cheese with
garlic and herbs, softened**
1 tablespoon all-purpose flour
¼ cup shredded carrots
¼ cup coarsely chopped walnuts
2 tablespoons chopped fresh parsley

Coating:
2 tablespoons chopped parsley
⅓ cup fine dry bread crumbs
2 tablespoons grated parmesan cheese
**2 tablespoons butter or
margarine, melted**

Place 1 chicken breast half, boned side up, between 2 pieces of clear plastic wrap. Pound lightly with flat side of mallet to form a 5½" square. Remove plastic. Repeat with remaining breast halves.

Stuffing:
In small mixer bowl, beat together the boursin cheese and flour until smooth. Stir in carrots, walnuts, and parsley. Place one-quarter of the cheese mixture on each chicken breast half. To roll up chicken, fold in 2 of the sides, then roll up jellyroll style. Press edges to seal.

Coating:
Stir parsley, bread crumbs and grated parmesan cheese in a small bowl. Brush chicken bundles with melted butter; roll in the coating mixture. Place seam side down, on a wire rack in 8" x 8" x 2" baking dish. Sprinkle the bundles with any remaining coating mixture. Bake in 350 degree oven for 40-45 minutes or until chicken is tender enough to be pierced with a fork and the coating mixture is golden.

Light Chicken Parisienne

4 servings.

4 teaspoons corn oil margarine
¼ cup flour
1 cup defatted chicken stock
¾ cup nonfat milk
¼ teaspoon salt
Freshly ground black pepper
Dash garlic powder
½ cup nonfat plain yogurt
½ cup sherry
2 whole chicken breasts, halved, skin removed
Pepper to taste
1 small onion chopped
1 cup sliced mushrooms

Melt margarine in skillet. Add flour and stir over medium heat 1 minute. Do not brown. Add chicken stock and nonfat milk. Using wire whisk, stir over medium heat until mixture comes to a boil. Add salt, pepper and garlic powder. Continue to cook 1 minute more. Remove from heat and combine with yogurt and sherry.

Season chicken breasts with freshly ground black pepper. Brown chicken on both sides in non-stick skillet. Arrange chicken, onions and mushrooms in 2 quart baking dish. Pour sauce mixture over all. Bake in 400 degree oven for 40-50 minutes. Serve over rice.

§ *Calories: 310 Fat: 8.5gm Cholesterol: 86mg Sodium: 567mg*

Chicken Breasts with Apricots

4 servings.

4 chicken breasts, cut in half, skinned and boned (total of 8 pieces)
8 tablespoons ground walnuts
4 tablespoons butter
8 dried apricots, minced
4 tablespoons apricot preserves or apricot sauce
4 tablespoons water

Roll chicken in walnuts to cover. Melt butter in frying pan and saute chicken breasts 3 minutes on each side. Add the dried apricots, apricot preserves and water. Simmer 3-4 minutes more, until chicken breasts are completely cooked.

Three Cheeses
Stuffed Chicken Breasts

8 servings.

½ cup frozen chopped spinach,
loosely packed
½ cup ricotta cheese
¼ cup grated parmesan cheese
¼ cup cottage cheese
3 eggs, beaten
4 whole chicken breasts, boned,
but not skinned
½ cup butter, melted
1 teaspoon paprika
¼ teaspoon salt
¼ teaspoon white pepper

Yogurt Sauce:
6 tomatoes, chopped
¼ cup plain yogurt
½ ounce basil leaves, finely chopped
2 drops red wine vinegar
Dash salt
White pepper

Thaw spinach and drain thoroughly. Combine spinach, ricotta, parmesan and cottage cheeses and eggs. Gently stuff mixture under skin of each chicken breasts. Combine butter, paprika, garlic powder, salt and white pepper. Brush each chicken generously with butter topping.

Bake in 350 degree oven for 20-25 minutes. Let cool and cut in half. Chicken may also be served hot. Accompany with a bowl of Yogurt Sauce.

Yogurt Sauce:
Combine tomatoes, yogurt and basil. Add vinegar, salt and pepper to taste.

Spicy Chicken Vegetable Micro

4 servings.

4 boneless, skinless chicken breast halves (about 6 ounces each), rinsed well and cut into 1″ cubes
1 large onion, coarsely chopped
3 garlic cloves, minced
1½ cups chicken broth
½ cup dry white wine
½ teaspoon tabasco sauce
3 medium carrots, trimmed, peeled and cut into sticks 2″ x ¼″ x ¼″
1 stalk celery, sliced ½″ thick
1 tablespoon cornstarch
1 cup fresh, canned or frozen peas
½ cup finely chopped parsley or
1 teaspoon dried rosemary
¼ teaspoon salt
¼ teaspoon black pepper

In 2 quart microwave-safe casserole, place chicken, onion, garlic, chicken broth, wine, tabasco sauce, carrots and celery. Cover and cook on high (100%) power 15 minutes or until meat and vegetables are tender, stirring once. Uncover. Dissolve cornstarch in ¼ cup cooking liquid. Add to chicken mixture and stir thoroughly until blended. Add peas, parsley and rosemary. Cover. Cook on high power 3 minutes or until sauce has thickened. Remove from oven. Season to taste with salt, pepper and additional tabasco sauce as desired.

Kung Pao Chicken with Broccoli

2 servings.

3 tablespoons water
2 tablespoons soy sauce
1 tablespoon corn starch
1 tablespoon dry sherry
1 teaspoon sugar
2 boneless chicken breast halves, skinned and cubed
1 tablespoon cornstarch
4 tablespoons peanut oil
¼ teaspoon dried red pepper flakes (optional)
5 green onions, chopped
2 garlic cloves, minced
1 teaspoon fresh ginger, peeled and minced
3 cups small broccoli florets
½ cup salted peanuts

Blend first 5 ingredients in bowl for sauce and set aside. Toss chicken with 1 tablespoon cornstarch to coat.

Heat 2 tablespoons oil in wok or heavy skillet over high heat. Add pepper flakes and blacken for 1 minute. Add chicken and cook until browned, stirring frequently for 1-2 minutes. Remove chicken using slotted spoon. Set aside. Add remaining 2 tablespoons oil to wok. Add onions, garlic and ginger and stir fry for 1 minute. Add broccoli and stir fry 2 minutes. Stir sauce and add to wok. Cover and cook until sauce is thickened and broccoli is crisp-tender, about 3 minutes. Mix in chicken and peanuts and heat through. Serve immediately with rice.

Monaco Chicken

6 servings.

**6 chicken breasts, halved,
skinned and boned
2 egg whites, lightly beaten
¾ cup seasoned bread crumbs
2-3 teaspoons olive oil
3 ounces skimmed
mozzarella cheese, sliced
1 tablespoon cornstarch
1½ cups low fat milk
¼ cup freshly grated parmesan cheese
2 tablespoons chopped parsley
⅛ teaspoon ground black pepper**

Dip chicken breasts into beaten egg whites and coat with bread crumbs. Heat half of the oil in skillet over medium heat. Add half of the chicken breasts. Brown lightly on both sides. Remove and place in baking dish. Heat other half of oil in skillet and repeat with remaining chicken. In a casserole dish, arrange chicken breasts in a single layer. Top breasts with mozzarella cheese.

Dissolve cornstarch in 3 tablespoons milk. Heat remaining milk, parmesan cheese, parsley and pepper in saucepan. Add cornstarch and stir until thickened. Pour over chicken and bake in 350 degree oven for 25-30 minutes.

Note: May be prepared ahead, refrigerated and baked about 30-35 minutes.

Baked Stuffed Chicken Breasts

6 servings.

6 chicken breasts, skinned and boned
6 pieces Monterey Jack cheese,
3″ x 1½″ thick
6 tablespoons chopped green chiles
¼ cup melted butter
1 cup seasoned bread crumbs
½ cup grated parmesan cheese

Flatten each chicken breast between saran wrap with a meat pounder until uniformly thin. Place 1 piece of Monterey Jack cheese and 1 tablespoon chopped chiles in the center of each chicken breast. Roll each stuffed breast carefully using a toothpick to hold together if necessary.

Combine bread crumbs and parmesan cheese in a shallow bowl. Dip chicken in melted butter, then coat with crumb mixture. Place in pyrex baking dish so chicken breasts are not touching. Preheat oven to 400 degrees. Bake uncovered for 30 minutes.

Cluck-Cluck Squares

4 to 6 servings.

4 chicken breast halves
2 tablespoons melted margarine
8 ounces cream cheese
¼ teaspoon salt
⅛ teaspoon pepper
2 tablespoons milk
1 tablespoon minced onion
1 8 ounce can refrigerated
quick crescent rolls
¼ teaspoon poultry seasoning
1 10.5 ounce can cream of
chicken soup
¼ cup milk

Stew chicken breasts. After cooking, remove skin and bones, cut chicken into small pieces. Blend margarine with cream cheese until smooth. Add chicken, salt, pepper, milk and onion. Mix well. Separate rolls into triangles. Place spoonful of chicken mixture into center of each triangle and pinch ends together to seal. Place on ungreased cookie sheet and bake in 350 degree oven for 20 minutes or until golden brown.

Combine soup and milk and heat thoroughly, stirring occasionally to make gravy. Serve chicken squares with gravy.

Mediterranean Chicken

4 servings.

4 whole skinned chicken breasts,
halved or 8 whole skinned chicken legs
1 large red onion, finely sliced
2 14 ounce cans whole Italian plum
tomatoes, drained
⅓ cup chicken broth
2 garlic cloves, mashed
½ teaspoon dried basil
½ teaspoon oregano
¼ teaspoon thyme
1 bay leaf, finely crumbled
¼ teaspoon fennel seed
Freshly ground pepper
¼ cup grated parmesan cheese

Place all ingredients, except cheese, in Dutch oven or large skillet. Cover and simmer for 45 minutes or until chicken is done. Chicken is done if juices run clear when meat is pierced deeply with a fork. Sprinkle with parmesan just before serving.

§ *Calories: 250 Fat: 5.5gm Cholesterol: 88mg Sodium: 565mg*

Chicken Florentine

6 servings.

2 10 ounce packages frozen
chopped spinach
3 whole chicken breasts, skinned,
boned and quartered
¼ pound butter, melted
½ cup flour
Salt, pepper and paprika
1½ cups whipping cream
⅓ cup grated parmesan cheese

Cook spinach according to package directions. Drain well and place in bottom of buttered baking dish (7″ x 11″). Dredge chicken pieces in melted butter, then flour. Lay chicken pieces in a single layer over spinach. Sprinkle with salt, pepper and paprika. Pour whipping cream over chicken. Sprinkle with parmesan cheese. Bake in preheated 400 degree oven for 20 minutes. Do not overcook.

Chicken Lasagna Florentine

12 servings.

1 dozen lasagna noodles
4 chicken breasts
1 10 ounce package frozen chopped spinach
1 small onion, chopped
1 clove garlic, minced
¼ pound mushrooms, sliced
2 tablespoons butter or margarine
2 10.37 ounce cans cream of chicken soup
1 pint sour cream
½ cup sherry or white wine
¼ cup parsley
Salt and pepper
1 pound mozzarella cheese, grated
1 cup grated parmesan cheese

Cook noodles and drain. Cook chicken and dice into ½" pieces. Defrost spinach, drain well. Saute onion, garlic and mushrooms in butter. Combine soup, sour cream and wine. To soup mixture add the onions, mushrooms, parsley, salt and pepper to taste, spinach and chicken pieces. Blend well.

In a 9" x 13" pan, layer 4 lasagna noodles, then one-third of the sauce and cheeses. Repeat 2 more times. Bake, uncovered, in 350 degree oven for 40 minutes.

Japanese Fried Chicken

4 servings.

4 tablespoons soy sauce
1 tablespoon sugar
2 tablespoons sake (rice wine)
1½ pounds chicken breast, boned and cut into 1" pieces
Vegetable oil for deep-frying
3 tablespoons cornstarch

Mix together the soy sauce and sugar until sugar is dissolved. Stir in sake. In a large bowl marinate chicken in mixture for about 1 hour.

In a pan, heat oil 3" deep to approximately 350 degrees. Remove the chicken from the marinade and coat with cornstarch. Deep fry chicken until crispy and browned, turning occasionally to ensure even cooking, about 5 minutes. Drain on rack or paper toweling and serve.

Chicken & Spinach

4 servings.

4 chicken breasts
1 chicken bouillon cube
1 package frozen spinach
1 can cream of chicken soup
1 cup grated cheddar cheese
½ cup mayonnaise
3 teaspoons lemon juice
½ cup bread crumbs (optional)

Place chicken in roaster and cover with water. Dissolve bouillon cube in the water. Cover and cook for 1 hour in 325 degree oven. Cool. Skin and bone chicken and cut into pieces.

Cook spinach and drain well. Layer spinach in bottom of casserole dish. Arrange chicken over spinach. Mix soup, cheese, mayonnaise and lemon juice together and spoon over chicken and spinach. Top with bread crumbs if desired. Bake for 40 minutes or until bubbly.

French Turkey Casserole

10 to 12 servings.

2½ cups coarse bread crumbs
1½ cup shredded Swiss cheese
½ cup chopped walnuts
¼ cup melted butter or margarine
½ teaspoon dried dill weed
4 cups cooked turkey chunks
2 cups cooked turkey ham chunks
1 cup chopped onions
¼ cup butter or margarine
⅓ cup flour
¾ cups half and half
1 tablespoon Dijon mustard
⅛ teaspoon ground nutmeg

Combine bread crumbs, ½ cup cheese, walnuts, melted butter and ¼ teaspoon dill weed. Set aside. Layer turkey, remaining cheese and turkey ham in 9″ x 13″ pan. Saute onions in butter, then stir in flour and blend in half and half. Add mustard, remaining dill and nutmeg. Bring to boil, stirring until thickened. Pour over ham and cover with reserved bread crumb mixture. Bake in 350 degree oven for 30 minutes.

Turkey Divine

6 to 8 servings.

½ cup sliced celery
¼ cup sliced almonds
1 4 ounce can sliced water chestnuts
1 tablespoon butter or margarine
2 cups cooked white rice
12-16 slices roasted turkey
2 cups turkey gravy or
2 cups cream of celery soup
½ cup cornflake crumbs or
Chinese noodles

Saute the celery, almonds and water chestnuts in butter until slightly browned. Combine with the cooked rice. Place rice mixture in a buttered baking dish.

Arrange turkey slices on top of rice mixture. Pour the gravy over turkey. Sprinkle cornflake crumbs over top and bake in 350 degree oven for 30 minutes or until thoroughly heated.

Turkey Schnitzel

6 servings.

6 turkey breast cutlets
2 eggs, lightly beaten
1 cup dry bread crumbs or
½ cup crumbs and ½ cup grated
parmesan cheese
2 tablespoons butter
2 tablespoons oil
¼ cup butter
¼ cup lemon juice
2 tablespoons chopped parsley

Flatten turkey cutlets to ¼″ thickness by pounding between 2 sheets of plastic wrap. Dip cutlets in eggs, then in bread crumbs or combined crumbs and cheese. Refrigerate 15 minutes.

Heat butter and oil and saute cutlets for 3 minutes on each side; remove to warmed platter. Add ¼ cup butter, lemon juice and parsley to skillet; bring to boil. Reduce slightly and pour over cutlets. Serve with noodles or spaetzle.

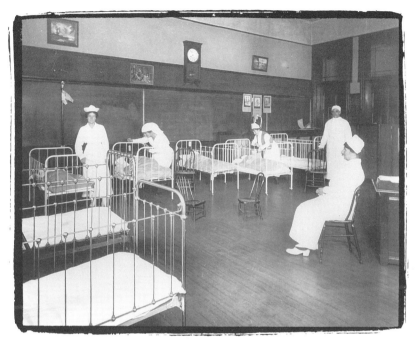

The new Children's Ward, circa 1914

beef, pork, veal and lamb

Roast Beef Pie with Potato Crust

When you have a cold roast of beef, cut as much as will half fill a baking dish suited to the size of your family; put this sliced beef into a stewpan with any gravy that you may have also saved, a lump of butter, a sliced onion and a seasoning of pepper and salt, with enough water to make plenty of gravy; thicken it, too, by dredging in a tablespoon of flour; cover it up on the fire, where it may stew gently, but not in danger of burning. Meanwhile there must be a sufficient quantity of potatoes to fill up your baking dish, after the stewed meat has been transferred to it. The potatoes must be boiled some, mashed smooth, and beaten up with milk and butter, as if they were to be served, and placed in a thick layer on top of the meat. Brush it over with egg, place the dish in oven, and let it remain there with beef, that the dish be not dry and tasteless. Serve with it tomato sauce, Worcestershire sauce or any other kind that you prefer. A good, plain dish.

The White House Cookbook © 1887

Easy Oven Stew

6 servings.

¼ cup flour
2 teaspoons salt
¼ teaspoon pepper
¼ teaspoon paprika
2 pounds boneless beef chuck or beef round, cut in 1" cubes
2 tablespoons oil
4 small onions, quartered
4 small carrots, pared and cut into 1" pieces
4 small potatoes, pared and halved
1 cup sliced celery
1 cup water
2 8 ounce cans tomato sauce with mushrooms

Combine flour, salt, pepper and paprika in paper bag. Drop in beef, a portion at a time; shake until coated. Mix beef with oil in 3 quart casserole. Bake in 400 degree oven for 30 minutes. Stir once. Add vegetables, water and tomato sauce. Mix well. Cover and bake in 350 degree oven for 1 hour 45 minutes or until done.

Sir Sydney's Skirt Steak

6 servings.

6 skirt steaks, trimmed of fat
¼ cup canola oil
½ cup light soy sauce
½ cup rice vinegar
¼ cup orange juice
½ cup pineapple juice
1 medium onion, coarsely chopped
¼ cup English mustard

Place skirt steaks in non-aluminum pan in single layer. Combine oil, soy sauce, vinegar, orange juice, pineapple juice, onion and mustard. Pour mixture over steaks. Marinate 12-24 hours.

Remove from marinade and cook steaks over medium-low coals or under broiler 4" from source of heat to desired doneness or medium rare for tender results.

Devilish Beef Ribs
with Mustard Sauce

6 to 8 servings.

8 pounds cooked beef ribs
(from prime rib of beef)
Salt
Pepper
¼ cup virgin olive oil
1 cup Dijon mustard
2½ cups plain, fresh breadcrumbs
10 ounces veal or beef stock
½ cup Madeira
½ teaspoon cornstarch
½ teaspoon water
2 tablespoons butter

Lightly season ribs with salt and pepper. Combine 3 tablespoons olive oil and all but 3 tablespoons mustard, blending well. Brush ribs lightly with mustard mixture. Dredge each rib in breadcrumbs and place on jellyroll pan. Sprinkle bones lightly with additional olive oil. Bake at 375 degrees until golden brown.

Combine stock and Madeira. Reduce by half. Combine cornstarch with water until smooth. Stir into sauce and cook until sauce coats back of spoon. Continue to simmer several minutes to blend flavors over low heat. Add butter and 3 tablespoons reserved mustard. Stir until smooth. Serve with ribs.

Italian Meatballs

6 servings.

2 eggs
2 tablespoons chopped parsley
½ cup seasoned bread crumbs
½ cup milk
¼ cup grated romano cheese
1 pound lean ground beef
½ pound ground pork
2 cloves garlic, minced or chopped
Salt and pepper

Beat eggs in bowl, add parsley. In another bowl, place bread crumbs and cover with milk—bread crumbs will absorb milk. Add cheese to egg mixture, then add bread crumbs, meat, garlic, salt and pepper. Mix well. Form into balls.

Fry in skillet over medium heat until brown on all sides. Meatballs are now ready to simmer in tomato sauce or to be frozen. If meatballs are made smaller, they are tasty appetizers.

Apple Pot Roast

8 servings.

2 tablespoons salad oil
4 pounds beef chuck roast
1 teaspoon salt
½ teaspoon dry basil
½ teaspoon ground ginger
¼ teaspoon ground cloves
¼ teaspoon pepper
1 bay leaf
½ cup dry white wine
¾ cup apple juice
1 large onion, coarsely chopped
2 tablespoons cornstarch,
blended with
2 tablespoons water
4 large tart apples, peeled, cored and
cut into eighths
Hot buttered noodles

In a 5 quart Dutch oven, heat oil over medium high heat. Add meat and brown well on both sides. Reduce heat and add salt, basil, ginger, cloves, pepper, bay leaf, wine, apple juice and onion. Bring to a boil, reduce heat and simmer covered, about 2 hours, or until meat is fork tender. Remove meat to a rimmed platter and keep warm.

Skim fat from pan juices. Blend cornstarch mixture into the juices and cook, stirring, over medium heat until thickened. Add apples, cover and simmer until fork tender, about 10-15 minutes. Pour apples and sauce over meat and serve with hot buttered noodles.

Fried Flank Steak

6 to 8 servings.

2 pounds flank steak, tenderized once by butcher (or cube steak)
½ cup brown sugar
½ cup soy sauce
1 teaspoon garlic powder
1 teaspoon ground ginger
5 eggs, beaten
1 bunch green onion tops, chopped
Cornstarch
Oil

Cut into bite-size pieces. In large bowl, stir together brown sugar, soy sauce, garlic powder and ginger. Add flank steak and marinate 15 minutes.

Combine eggs and green onions in medium bowl. Place cornstarch in separate bowl. Dip each piece of meat lightly into cornstarch then dip into beaten eggs with green onion. Heat ½" oil in medium sized skillet. Fry meat in hot oil until golden brown, turning once. Drain on paper towels and serve.

Orange Ginger Beef with Vegetables

4 to 5 servings

1 pound beef (top sirloin steak), well trimmed and cut into 1" strips
4 tablespoons soy sauce
½ teaspoon ground ginger
1-2 teaspoons shredded orange peel
1 tablespoon vegetable oil
2 cups broccoli florets
1 small red pepper, cut into thin strips
⅔ cups picante sauce
½ teaspoon sugar
3 green onions, sliced diagonally
⅓ cup orange juice
2 tablespoons cornstarch
2 cups cooked rice

Toss meat strips with soy sauce, ginger and orange peel. Set aside for 10 minutes.

Heat oil in wok or 10" skillet. Stir fry meat mixture over medium heat until it is no longer pink. Remove and serve. Add broccoli, red pepper, picante sauce, sugar and onion. Cook about 3 minutes. Return meat to wok.

Combine orange juice and cornstarch and add. Cook and stir 1 minute or until thickened. Serve over rice.

§ *Calories: 398 Fat 11.2gm Cholesterol: 73mg Sodium:1237mg*

Mozzarella Beef Roll

6 to 8 servings.

⅓ pound lean ground beef
½ teaspoon salt
¼ teaspoon pepper
½ cup bread crumbs
1 tablespoon onion flakes
1 egg, slightly beaten
1 8 ounce can mushrooms, stems and pieces
1½ cups grated mozzarella cheese
1 15 ounce can tomato sauce
3 tablespoons dry vermouth

Combine meat, salt, pepper, bread crumbs, onion flakes and egg. Mix thoroughly. Drain mushrooms, reserving juice and set aside. Add enough liquid to mushroom juice to make ¾ cup. Add to meat mixture.

On foil or wax paper, press meat into a 14″ x 10″ rectangle. Sprinkle with cheese leaving a ½″ border. Roll up jellyroll fashion beginning with 1 short side. Place seam side down in 9″ x 13″ pan.

Combine tomato sauce with vermouth, spread half of sauce over roll. Bake in 375 degree oven for 50 minutes. Drain any grease. Combine remaining sauce with mushrooms and spread over roll. Bake 15 minutes longer.

Grilled Mustard Ribs

4 servings.

4 pounds beef ribs cut into separate ribs
1 cup Dijon mustard
1 cup dry white wine
2 tablespoons salad oil
2 tablespoons honey
2 teaspoons dry tarragon
2 cloves garlic, pressed or minced

Place ribs in large plastic bag. Mix remaining ingredients and pour marinade over ribs and seal bag. Mix to coat and put in a 9″ x 13″ pan. Chill, turning meat occasionally, at least 4 hours or overnight.

Place meat on grill 4″-6″ above a solid bed of medium hot coals. Cook, turning and basting until browned, but still slightly pink near bone, about 15-20 minutes.

Sauerbraten

6 to 8 servings.

3-4 pounds beef blade pot roast
1 clove garlic, halved
2 teaspoons salt
¼ teaspoon pepper
2 cups cider vinegar
2 cups water
2 onions, sliced
2 bay leaves
1 teaspoon peppercorns
¼ cup sugar
2 tablespoons margarine

Gingersnap Gravy:
¾ cup crushed gingersnaps
1 tablespoon sugar
Cooking liquid from roast

Rub meat with cut surface of garlic, then with salt and pepper. Place meat and garlic into a deep casserole. Heat the vinegar, water, onions, bay leaves, peppercorns and sugar just until boiling; pour over meat and allow to cool. Cover and refrigerate 4 days, turning meat each day.

Remove meat; strain and reserve liquid for cooking the meat. Brown meat in heated margarine in a Dutch oven, turning to brown evenly. Add half of the reserved liquid; cover and simmer 2-3 hours or until meat is tender, adding additional liquid as needed. Slice meat; serve with Gingersnap Gravy, if desired.

Gingersnap Gravy:
In Dutch oven stir gingersnaps and sugar into cooking liquid. Simmer 10 minutes, stirring occasionally.

Bev's Barbecued Brisket

6 to 8 servings.

1 piece 3-3½ pounds center-cut
fresh beef brisket
1 medium-sized onion, finely chopped
½ cup catsup
2 teaspoons horseradish
½ teaspoon whole cloves
1 cinnamon stick, about 2"
2 tablespoons brown sugar,
firmly packed
⅓ cup water
⅓ cup dry white wine
Unsalted meat tenderizer

Trim and discard surface fat from brisket. Put meat in a plastic bag, about 4 quart size; add onion, catsup, horseradish, cloves, cinnamon, vinegar, brown sugar, water and wine. Seal bag and rotate to mix well. Set bag in a pan and chill for at least 2 hours or up to 1 day.

Lift brisket from bag and pour marinade into 1-1½ quart pan. Pat meat and apply tenderizer according to package directions. Place meat on a lightly greased grill 4"-6" above a solid bed of low coals. Cook, turning often, until a meat thermometer inserted in thickest part registers 135-140 degrees for rare to medium-rare, 25-30 minutes.

Transfer meat to a carving board, drape with foil and let stand for 10 minutes for juices to settle.

Top Hat Pork Chops

4 servings.

4 ¾"-1" thick pork chops (loin cut)
1 15 ounce can creamed corn
Italian bread crumbs
Salt and pepper

Trim pork chops of excess fat. Mix creamed corn with enough bread crumbs to make a thick mixture. Salt and pepper to taste. Divide this mixture on each chop. Put a small piece of the fat from the chops on top of each corn mixture. Use a broiler pan to bake the chops in 350 degree oven for about 1 hour.

Pork Chops with a Delicate Sweet-Sour Sauce

6 servings.

¼ cup black currant preserves
1½ tablespoons prepared Dijon-style mustard
6 center-cut pork chops, 1"-1½" thick
Salt and freshly ground pepper to taste
Watercress (garnish)

Sauce:
Cooking liquid from pork chops
⅓ cup white wine vinegar

Mix the preserves and mustard together in a small bowl. Set aside.

Heat a nonstick skillet just large enough to hold the pork chops comfortably, and brown them lightly on both sides. Season with salt and pepper to taste and spoon the currant and mustard mixture evenly over them. Cover pork chops, reduce heat and cook for 20 minutes, or until the chops are done. Transfer them to a platter and keep them warm in the oven.

Sauce:
Remove excess fat from the skillet. Add the vinegar, set pan over medium heat and bring juices to a boil, stirring and scraping up any brown bits. When the sauce is reduced by about one third, pour it over the chops and serve immediately, garnished with watercress.

Chinese Style Country Ribs

6 to 8 servings.

¼ cup soy sauce
¼ cup orange marmalade
2 tablespoons catsup
1 clove garlic, crushed
3-4 pounds country style spareribs

Combine soy sauce, marmalade, catsup and garlic. Brush on both sides of ribs. Place ribs in a slow-cooking pot. Pour remaining sauce over ribs. Cover and cook on low for 8-10 hours.

Sweet & Sour Pork

6 servings.

1½ pounds pork tenderloin,
cut into 1″-2″ strips
2 tablespoons shortening
1 cup water
1 chicken bouillon cube
¼ teaspoon salt
1 20.5 ounce can pineapple chunks
¼ cup brown sugar
2 tablespoons cornstarch
¼ cup vinegar
1 tablespoon soy sauce
1 medium green pepper, cut in strips
¼ cup thinly sliced onion

Brown pork in 2 tablespoons shortening. Stir in 1 cup water, chicken bouillon cube and salt. Cover and simmer until tender, about 20-25 minutes.

Drain pineapple, reserving syrup. Combine brown sugar, cornstarch, pineapple syrup, vinegar and soy sauce. Cook and stir until bubbly. Add sauce to pork. Stir in pineapple, green pepper and onion. Cook 2-3 minutes and serve over steamed rice.

§ *Calories: 239 Fat: 6.6gm Cholesterol: 44mg Sodium: 424mg*

Ham Maple Bake

2 servings.

1 ham slice, 1¼″-1½″ thick
Cloves
1 cup maple syrup

Trim excess fat from ham. Stud meat with cloves every 2″. Place in greased baking dish, same size as ham slice. Pour syrup over ham. Bake, uncovered, in a 300 degree oven for 45 minutes-1 hour, or until tender. Baste occasionally.

Wine Poached Sausages & Fettucini

6 servings.

2 pounds sweet Italian sausages
2 cups dry red wine
3 cups sliced green onions
2½ tablespoons olive oil
⅔ cup chopped sun dried tomatoes packed in olive oil
⅓ cup golden raisins
½ tablespoon fresh marjoram or ½ teaspoon dried
12 ounces fettucine, cooked al dente

Pierce sausages. In saucepan just large enough to hold sausages in one layer, simmer in wine until firm to the touch—about 10 minutes. Drain sausages, reserving wine. Set sausages aside. Saute onion in 2 tablespoons olive oil, about 5 minutes. Skim fat from wine, puree tomato with wine. When onion is soft, add puree, raisins and marjoram. Simmer until sauce coats back of spoon—about 5 minutes. While sauce is simmering, finish cooking sausages by grilling in ½ tablespoon oil until browned.

Toss fettucini with sauce. Divide pasta and sausages among plates. Garnish with fresh marjoram.

Veal Scaloppine

4 servings.

2 pounds veal, thinly sliced
Salt and pepper
2 tablespoons flour
2 tablespoons Canola oil
3 ounces sliced mushrooms
1 medium green pepper, cooked and peeled
1 cup sherry or Marsala wine
2 tablespoons water
2 tablespoons tomato sauce

Cut veal in 5″ squares, very thin slices. Season with salt and pepper. Flour lightly. Heat oil and brown veal well on both sides. Add mushrooms and green pepper. Add sherry. Simmer 3 minutes longer. Add water and tomato sauce. Simmer for 5 minutes.

Veal with Peppers

4 servings.

1 pound veal scallopini
¾ cup white wine Worcestershire sauce
2 tablespoons oil
1 large green pepper, cut in thin strips
1 tablespoon cornstarch

Cut veal into 2″ x 1″ slices. Place in mixing bowl with 2 tablespoons white wine Worcestershire sauce and toss to coat meat. Set aside 5 minutes. Heat oil in skillet, add green pepper strips and saute 5 minutes. Add meat and brown. Mix cornstarch with remaining white wine Worcestershire sauce and add to pan. Cook until peppers are tender and sauce has thickened—about 4 minutes.

May use sliced chicken or turkey in place of the veal.

Deviled Veal Chops

2 servings.

1½ tablespoons Worcestershire sauce
⅛ teaspoon garlic powder
1 tablespoon Dijon mustard
1 teaspoon vegetable oil
5 5 ounce veal chops

Preheat broiler. Combine Worcestershire sauce, garlic powder, mustard and oil. Spread half of mixture on top of chops. With mixture side up, place veal on broiler pan. Broil 3″ from heat for 5 minutes. Turn veal. Spread with remaining mixture. Broil 5 minutes more.

Lemon Veal

4 servings.

1 tablespoon olive oil
1 pound veal, sliced very thin
Salt and pepper
½ cup water
Juice of 1 lemon
1 teaspoon cornstarch

Add olive oil to large frying pan. When hot, add veal seasoned with salt and pepper. Fry quickly on both sides. Remove veal from pan and add ½ cup water or more plus juice from lemon. Put veal back in pan. Cover and simmer for 15-20 minutes.

To make gravy, combine cornstarch with a little water and blend well. Slowly add to veal and adjust seasonings as desired. Serve on hot platter.

§ *Calories: 211 Fat: 9.3gm Cholesterol: 107mg Sodium: 154mg*

Veal a La Suisse

6 servings.

2 pounds veal, thinly sliced
½ cup butter
3 tablespoons sherry or Marsala wine
1 tablespoon flour
1 bouillon cube
½ cup water
½ cup milk
¼ teaspoon nutmeg
Freshly ground black pepper
½ pound Swiss cheese, sliced

Pound veal lightly until thin. Heat 6 tablespoons of butter in skillet. Add veal and brown lightly on both sides. Add wine and cool a few seconds. Transfer veal to a baking dish. Melt remaining butter in sauce pan and add flour—whisk until blended. Dissolve bouillon cube in boiling water and add milk. Add to butter/flour mixture, whisking until smooth. Add nutmeg and pepper. Arrange veal in a single layer. Top with sauce and arrange cheese over all. Heat under broiler until cheese melts.

Blue Cheese Lamb Chops

2 servings.

2 loin lamb chops, each cut 1½″ thick
1 ounce blue cheese
2 teaspoons Worcestershire sauce

Heat broiler. With small sharp knife, trim fat from chops and cut pocket in center of one side. Use half of the blue cheese to stuff each chop. Press to close pocket.

Place on broiler pan and sprinkle with Worcestershire sauce, using ½ teaspoon on each chop. Broil 7 minutes. Turn; sprinkle with remaining Worcestershire sauce and cook 7 minutes or until pink.

Lamb & White Wine Casserole

6 servings.

1 teaspoon salt
Freshly ground black pepper to taste
3 tablespoons flour
2 pounds shoulder of lamb, boned and cubed
2 tablespoons oil
4 cloves garlic, crushed
1 cup dry white wine
1 bay leaf
2 egg yolks
1 tablespoon lemon juice
2 tablespoons chopped parsley

Combine salt, pepper and flour. Coat lamb with seasoned flour and brown in oil and garlic. Place in casserole dish with wine and bay leaf, cover and bake for 1 hour at 300 degrees. Stir egg yolks and lemon juice into casserole and sprinkle with finely chopped parsley.

Colonial Lamb

6 to 8 servings.

Leg of lamb
Rosemary sprigs
½ teaspoon salt
Pepper
6-8 peach halves
½ cup peach syrup
1 teaspoon cinnamon
¼ teaspoon ground cloves
Mint jelly

Make several incisions in leg of lamb and insert small sprigs of rosemary. Sprinkle with salt and pepper and place lamb on a rack in a shallow roasting pan, inserting a meat thermometer so tip does not touch bone. Roast, uncovered, in 325 degree oven until meat thermometer registers 175-180 degrees. Drain syrup from peaches, retain ½ cup. Simmer syrup, vinegar and spices until reduced to half of volume, then add peach halves to heat through and coat with glaze. Surround cooled lamb with spiced peach halves. Fill depressions in peaches with mint jelly. Serve with new potatoes, peas and buttered cauliflower.

Lemon Mint Baskets

4 baskets.

4 lemons
1 12 ounce jar apple-mint jelly

Insert 2 toothpicks, ¼″ apart in center of lemon. With a sharp knife, cut lemon halfway, on each side of toothpick, to make handle. On each side, cut away top half of lemon. Scoop out pulp from under handle and form inside basket. Fill 'baskets' with apple-mint jelly.

Continental Lamb Shanks

6 servings.

⅓ cup flour
Salt and pepper to taste
6 lamb shanks
¼ cup oil
1 large onion, chopped
3 tablespoons Worcestershire sauce
1 teaspoon basil
¾ cup dry white wine
2 cans (8 ounces each) tomato sauce with mushrooms
3 tablespoons chopped parsley

Combine flour, salt and pepper. Coat lamb shanks with flour mixture. In a large skillet, heat oil, add lamb shanks and brown. Add remaining ingredients. Cover and simmer 1 hour 30 minutes or until tender. Skim off fat. Arrange meat on deep platter. Pour sauce over.

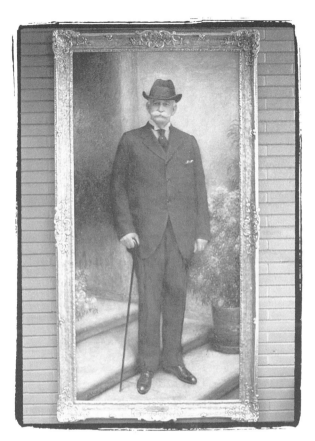

Henry E. Huntington, hospital benefactor

sauces

Bechamel Sauce

Put three tablespoonfuls of butter in a saucepan; and three tablespoonfuls of nutmeg, ten peppercorns, a teaspoonful of salt; beat all well together; then add to this three slices of onion, two slices of carrot, two sprigs of parsley, two of thyme, a bay leaf and half a dozen mushrooms cut up. Moisten the whole with a pint of stock or water and a cup of sweet cream. Set it on the stove and cook slowly for half an hour, watching closely that it does not burn; then strain through a sieve. Most excellent with roast veal, meats and fish.

The White House Cookbook ©1887

❧

Citrus Cream Sauce
for Fish or Vegetables

2 cups.

2 whole oranges
1 whole lemon
2 eggs
1 cup dairy sour cream
Salt
Cayenne pepper to taste

Grate colored portion of peel from oranges and lemon. Then, squeeze fruit to get juice. (Discard pitch.) In top of double boiler, combine grated peel and juices with eggs and sour cream; beat well.

Set over simmering water and, while stirring, cool until slightly thickened. Remove from heat and keep warm. Season to taste with salt and cayenne pepper. Serve over cooked fish or vegetables.

Cranberry Chutney

5 to 6 cups.

1 pound cranberries
1 cup granulated sugar
½ cup brown sugar
½ cup golden raisins
2 teaspoons ground cinnamon
½ teaspoon ground cloves
1½ teaspoons ground ginger
¼ teaspoon ground allspice
1 cup water
1 cup baking apples, peeled and chopped
½ cup celery, chopped

Simmer cranberries, sugars, raisins, spices, and water in an uncovered 2 quart saucepan over medium heat. Stir frequently until juice is released from berries, approximately 15 minutes. Reduce heat, stir in apples and celery. Simmer uncovered until thick, approximately 15 minutes. Cool. May be poured into jars to give as gifts or left in one large container for a buffet.

Chow-Chow Relish

4 pints.

1 quart cabbage, chopped
(about 1 small head)
3 cups cauliflower, chopped
(about 1 medium head)
2 cups onion, chopped
2 cups green tomatoes, chopped
(about 4 medium)
2 cups green peppers, chopped
(about 4 medium)
1 cup sweet red pepper, chopped
(about 2 medium)
3 tablespoons salt
2½ cups vinegar
1½ cups sugar
2 teaspoons dry mustard
1 teaspoon turmeric
½ teaspoon ginger
2 teaspoons celery seeds
1 teaspoon mustard seeds

Combine chopped cabbage, cauliflower, onions, green tomatoes, green and red peppers and sprinkle with salt. Let stand 4-6 hours in cool place. Drain well.

Combine vinegar, sugar, dry mustard, turmeric, ginger, celery seeds and mustard seeds. Simmer 10 minutes. Add vegetables and simmer for 10 minutes. Bring to a boil. Pack boiling hot mixture into hot sterilized jars, leaving ⅛″ head space. Process for 10 minutes in boiling hot water. Adjust caps.

Instant Hollandaise Sauce

6 servings.

1 cup mayonnaise
¼ cup lime juice
Salt and pepper to taste

Combine all ingredients in a small saucepan. Bring to a boil. Remove from heat; stir and pour over cooked vegetables.

Regular Creme Fraiche

1 cup.

1 cup heavy cream
2 tablespoons buttermilk

Shake well in covered glass jar. Put in warm place for 12 hours. Refrigerate.

Low-Cal Substitute Creme Fraiche

2 cups.

1¼ cups evaporated skim milk
1 cup plain non-fat yogurt
1½ teaspoons lemon juice

Combine all ingredients. Whisk thoroughly. Cover and let stand at room temperature at least six hours. Refrigerate.

§ *Calories: 22 Fat: 0.4gm Cholesterol: 5mg Sodium: 26mg*

Basic Pesto

1½ cups.

5 ounces basil leaves
¾ ounce garlic, peeled and crushed
¼ cup pine nuts
1 cup grated parmesan cheese
¼ teaspoon salt
1 cup olive oil

Insert metal blade in food processor container. Add basil and process until finely shredded. Add garlic, pine nuts, parmesan and salt. Add oil slowly through tube. Process to coarse paste.

Mandarin Pesto

1⅓ cups.

4 cups packed fresh spinach leaves
½ cup packed fresh basil
¼ cup packed fresh cilantro
¼ cup packed parsley
¼ cup sliced green onion
½ cup olive oil or cooking oil
2 tablespoons red wine vinegar
1 tablespoon sesame oil
1 tablespoon soy sauce
1 tablespoon oyster sauce
1 teaspoon grated fresh ginger root
1 teaspoon shredded orange peel
1 clove garlic
Several dashes bottled hot-pepper sauce

In a saucepan cook spinach, covered, in a small amount of boiling water 2-3 minutes; drain. Press out remaining moisture with paper towels. Place spinach and remaining ingredients in a food processor or blender and puree until smooth. Add a bit more oil, if necessary.

Serve with edible centerpiece of fresh vegetables.

Villa Romano Pesto

6 to 8 servings.

4 ounces basil leaves
2 cloves garlic, crushed
2 tablespoons lightly toasted pine nuts
½ cup extra virgin olive oil
1 teaspoon salt
½ cup grated parmesan cheese
2 tablespoons grated romano cheese
4 tablespoons butter
3-4 medium tomatoes, peeled and seeded
1 pound linguine

Insert metal blade in food processor container. Add basil, garlic, pine nuts, olive oil and salt. Process to coarse paste. Beat in cheeses and 3 tablespoons softened butter by hand. Mince tomatoes very fine. Cook linguine in boiling salted water until tender yet firm. Drain off all but 1 tablespoon cooking water. Add about 1 tablespoon butter.

For each serving, add half of a tomato to linguine then add 3-4 tablespoons pesto sauce. Toss quickly and serve at once.

Mabel's Hot & Sweet Mustard

4 cups.

1⅓ cups white wine vinegar or
champagne vinegar
1⅓ cups dry mustard
2 cups sugar
6 large eggs

In a small bowl, mix vinegar and dry mustard; let stand for 1 hour. Add sugar and eggs to mustard mixture; beat with whisk until smooth. Pour into a heavy 1½-2 quart pan. Stir with a whisk often over medium heat until mixture thickens and begins to bubble, 10-12 minutes. Remove from heat. Pour into jars. If made ahead, cool, cover and chill up to 3 months.

To seal, pour hot mustard into hot, clean sterilized jars to within ⅛" of top. Clean jar rim. Top with hot, clean canning lids. Let cool 24 hours. Press down on lid. If it stays down, jar is sealed; if it pops up, refrigerate as above. Store sealed jars in a cool, dry place up to 1 year.

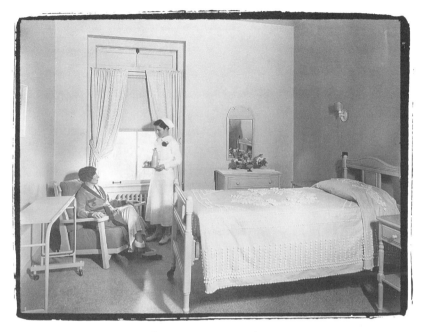

Patient room, circa 1940

vegetables, rice and pasta

Ladies Cabbage

Boil a firm white cabbage fifteen minutes, changing the water then for more

from the boiling tea-kettle. When tender, drain and set aside until perfectly cold. Chop

fine and add two beaten eggs, a tablespoonful of butter, pepper, salt, three tablespoons

full of rich milk or cream. Stir all well together, and bake in a buttered

pudding-dish until brown. Serve very hot. This dish resembles

cauliflower and is very digestible and palatable.

The White House Cookbook ©1887

Asparagus & Miso Sauce

4 servings.

1 pound asparagus
2 teaspoons salt
½ cup shiromiso (white soybean paste)
2 tablespoons Japanese rice vinegar
1½ tablespoons sugar
1 tablespoon mirin (sweet rice wine)
1 teaspoon freshly grated
Ginger root

Break off tough ends of asparagus and wash spears. Bring a generous amount of water and the salt to a boil and add the asparagus. Return to a boil, then turn off heat. Cover and let stand for 10 minutes. Drain and run cold water over asparagus to retain bright color.

Mix together remaining ingredients to make a soft paste. Serve in a little dish as a dipping sauce for asparagus or cut asparagus into 1½″ lengths, pour sauce over, toss and serve as a salad.

Green Beans Gratin

12 servings.

¾ cup diced onions
¼ cup olive oil
1 cup sliced mushrooms
1 teaspoon salt
¼ teaspoon pepper
3 cups fresh green beans
(about 1 ¼ pounds), trimmed and sliced
½ cup sour cream
¾ pound mozzarella cheese, shredded
½ cup grated parmesan cheese

In skillet, cook onions in oil over moderate heat for 5 minutes. Add the mushrooms, salt and pepper and cook 2 minutes, stirring constantly. Add green beans and cook mixture over low heat for 20 minutes. Transfer half the mixture to a buttered 10″ gratin dish and cover with sour cream. Top with remaining bean mixture, mozzarella and parmesan cheeses. Bake 20 minutes at 425 degrees or until cheeses are melted and bubbly.

Chilled Baby Lima Beans

4 servings.

1 10 ounce package
frozen baby lima beans
3 tablespoons chopped chives
1 small clove garlic, minced
⅛ teaspoon salt
¼ teaspoon pepper
½ cup sour cream
2 tablespoons chopped pimentos

Cook lima beans according to package directions. Drain. Toss beans with chives, garlic, salt, pepper and sour cream. Top with pimentos. Chill and serve.

Spanish Bean Pot

10 servings.

2 15 ounce cans red kidney beans
2 tablespoons bacon fat
1 clove garlic, minced
1 pinch thyme
1 pinch rosemary
1 small bay leaf
2 whole cloves
1 teaspoon salt
2 teaspoons dry mustard
½ teaspoon cayenne pepper
2 tablespoons cider vinegar
½ cup juice from pickled watermelon
1 onion, sliced very thin
4 slices bacon, cooked and crumbled
¼ cup strong coffee
1 ounce brandy

Put beans in pot. Mix together all other ingredients except onion, bacon, coffee and brandy. Pour mixture over beans, stir and bake 1 hour in 275 degree oven. Cover top with onion and then with bacon. Bake 5 minutes longer in 400 degree oven. Stir in coffee and brandy. Heat 5 more minutes.

Berry Berry Beets

6 servings.

1 16 ounce can whole berry or
   jellied cranberry sauce
2 tablespoons orange juice
1 teaspoon grated orange peel
   ⅛ teaspoon salt
2 cups cooked beets,
   drained and sliced

Place cranberry sauce in medium pan. Heat over moderate heat until it melts. Add orange juice, orange peel and salt. Mix well. Gently mix in beets. Heat until bubbly.

Beets & Pineapple

6 servings.

   ½ cup sugar
2 tablespoons cornstarch
   ¼ cup vinegar
Pineapple juice, drained from can
2 cans baby pickled beets drained or
   whole beets, quartered and drained
1 16 ounce can pineapple chunks or
   tidbits, drained

For sauce combine sugar, cornstarch, vinegar and pineapple juice. Cook until thick. Add beets and pineapple chunks. Heat through and serve.

Great side dish with ham, chicken or turkey.

German Red Cabbage

6 to 8 servings.

2 tablespoons butter
1 head red cabbage, chopped
1 small onion, chopped
1 large tart apple, chopped
4 tablespoons vinegar
3 tablespoons brown sugar
1-2 tablespoons water (if needed)
Salt and pepper

Heat butter and add cabbage, onion and apple. Cook slowly until onion is tender but not brown. Add vinegar, brown sugar and water, if needed. Cover and simmer for 20 minutes. Season to taste with salt and pepper.

§ *Calories: 115 Fat: 4.4gm Cholesterol: 10mg Sodium: 106mg*

Seasoned Carrot Bake

6 to 8 servings.

8 carrots, sliced
½ cup mayonnaise
1 tablespoon minced onion
1 tablespoon prepared horseradish
½ teaspoon salt
¼ teaspoon pepper
½ cup fine cracker crumbs
½ teaspoon paprika
¼ cup chopped fresh parsley

Cook carrots in enough water to cover until just tender. Drain, saving one-quarter of the cooking liquid. Place carrots in greased oven-proof serving dish.

In small bowl, combine reserved liquid with mayonnaise, onion, horseradish, salt and pepper. Spread over carrots. Sprinkle with cracker crumbs, paprika and parsley. Bake at 375 degrees, uncovered, for 15-20 minutes.

Sunshine Carrots

4 servings.

5 medium carrots, sliced
1 tablespoon sugar
1 teaspoon cornstarch
¼ teaspoon salt
¼ teaspoon ginger
¼ cup orange juice
1 teaspoon vinegar
2 tablespoons butter
Chopped parsley (optional)

Cook sliced carrots in boiling salted water until tender and drain. Combine dry ingredients in saucepan. Add orange juice and vinegar. Cook until thickened and bubbly. Boil for 1 minute. Stir in butter and pour over hot carrots. Sprinkle with chopped parsley if desired.

§ *Calories: 112 Fat: 5.9gm Cholesterol: 16mg Sodium: 237mg*

Cheesy Cauliflower Casserole

6 servings.

19 ounces fresh or thawed cauliflorets
½ cup nonfat milk
3 eggs
1 teaspoon cornstarch
1 teaspoon spicy mustard
Dash hot pepper sauce
3 tablespoons grated parmesan cheese
3 tablespoons seasoned bread crumbs

Arrange cauliflower in baking dish. Beat milk, eggs, cornstarch, mustard and hot pepper sauce until well mixed. Pour over cauliflower. Sprinkle with cheese and bread crumbs and bake in 350 degree oven for about 30 minutes.

§ *Calories: 73 Fat: 3.2gm Cholesterol: 88mg Sodium: 116mg*

Gulliver's Creamed Corn

8 servings.

2 packages frozen corn or
20 ounces canned corn, drained
8 ounces whipping cream
8 ounces homogenized milk
1 teaspoon salt
¼ teaspoon accent (optional)
6 tablespoons sugar
Pinch of cayenne pepper
2 tablespoons melted butter
2 tablespoons flour

Combine first 7 ingredients in a pot and bring to a boil. Simmer 5 minutes. Blend butter with flour, add to the corn and mix well. Simmer for 2 minutes, then serve.

Chile Hominy Casserole

8 to 10 servings.

2 20 ounce cans hominy, drained
3 tablespoons chopped onion
1½ cups sour cream
1½ cups shredded
Monterey Jack cheese
4 ounces chopped Ortega chiles, drained
¾ teaspoon salt
½ cup finely crumbled bread crumbs

Combine all ingredients together, except bread crumbs. Put into a 2½ quart casserole dish and sprinkle with bread crumbs. Bake 30-40 minutes in 350 degree oven.

Grandmère Claudine's Stuffed Eggplant

4 to 6 servings.

2 medium eggplants
1 pound ground beef
1 small onion, chopped
½ cup minute rice
3 eggs
¾ cup parmesan cheese
Salt and pepper
Italian bread crumbs

Rinse eggplants, cut off blossom end, cut into quarters lengthwise and place them in a pan with water. Cook until the eggplants are parboiled. Drain in a colander to cool. When you are able to handle the quarter, scoop out the pulp and place in a bowl. Try not to rip the skins. Place the skins in a greased baking dish.

Rice the pulp with a potato ricer or chop the pulp in a food processor. Brown the ground beef and onions until the onions are soft. Remove the pan from the stove. Add the pulp from the eggplant and mix thoroughly. Add the rice, then the eggs one at a time. Lastly add the parmesan cheese, salt and pepper. Spoon the mixture onto the eggplant skins. Sprinkle with Italian bread crumbs on top. Bake in 350 degree oven for about 1 hour.

Mushroom Tart

4 to 6 servings.

½ cup finely chopped shallots
½ cup finely chopped onion
2 tablespoons butter
1 pound mushrooms, finely chopped
2 tablespoons flour
1 cup Creme Fraiche
3 egg yolks
½ teaspoon white pepper
1 teaspoon salt
1 teaspoon nutmeg
2 tablespoons parsley
Sour cream or Creme Fraiche
Chopped parsley

In large frying pan, saute shallots and onions in butter for 1 minute. Add mushrooms and saute over low heat until most of the mushroom liquid has evaporated (about 5 minutes). Sprinkle flour over mushroom mixture and blend in quickly. Add Creme Fraiche and stir to blend. Continue cooking over medium heat until mixture begins to boil. Remove from heat.

Beat egg yolks slightly and add 2 tablespoons of mushroom mixture. Whisk to combine. Quickly whisk egg combination into mushroom and onions. Combine quickly and thoroughly. Add white pepper, salt, nutmeg and parsley. Let cool.

Pour into glass pie plate and bake 25 minutes in 325 degree oven. Garnish with dollops of sour cream or Creme Fraiche and freshly chopped parsley.

Can be made ahead and frozen. Bake directly from freezer.

Herbed Potatoes

12 servings.

4 ounces margarine or butter, melted
2 packages onion soup mix
1 tablespoon rosemary
6 large baking potatoes, unpeeled, sliced thick

Combine all ingredients in large flat baking dish and mix together. Cover and bake in 350 degree oven for 1 hour.

Acadian Stuffed Mushrooms

6 servings.

8-12 **large mushrooms**
2 **tablespoons butter**
¼ **cup finely chopped onion**
1 **garlic clove, minced**
¼ **pound bulk pork sausage**
⅛ **teaspoon dried thyme**
1 **tablespoon chopped fresh parsley**
Pinch of ground allspice
Pinch of cayenne pepper
Pinch of hot dried red pepper flakes
Salt and pepper
Dash of liquid smoke
2 **tablespoons fresh**
French bread crumbs
2 **tablespoons grated parmesan cheese**
½ **teaspoon hot paprika**

Preheat oven to 400 degrees. Remove and chop mushroom stems, set caps aside. Melt butter, add and cook mushroom stems, onions and garlic until softened. Add sausage, thyme, parsley, allspice, cayenne pepper, red pepper, salt, pepper and liquid smoke.

Stuff mushroom caps with this mixture and arrange in oiled baking dish. Mix together bread crumbs, cheese and paprika. Sprinkle over stuffing. Bake for 20 minutes. Serve hot.

Tangy English Potatoes

6 servings.

6 **medium potatoes, peeled**
½ **cup butter**
2 **teaspoons Worcestershire sauce**
1 **teaspoon salt**
¼ **teaspoon paprika**

Cut potatoes into julienne strips. Boil in lightly salted water for 5 minutes. Drain.

Cover cookie sheet with aluminum foil. Arrange potatoes on sheet. Melt butter in small saucepan. Stir in Worcestershire sauce, salt and paprika. Heat thoroughly. Brush potatoes with sauce. Bake in 375 degree oven until brown and crisp, about 15-20 minutes.

Broccoli Stuffed Onions

3 servings.

3 medium onions
1 10 ounce package frozen chopped broccoli, cooked
½ cup grated parmesan cheese
⅓ cup mayonnaise
2 teaspoons lemon juice
2 tablespoons butter
2 tablespoons flour
¼ teaspoon salt
⅔ cup milk
1 3 ounce package cream cheese, cubed

Peel and cut onions in half. Parboil in salt water 10-12 minutes, then drain. Remove centers leaving ¾". Chop center portions to equal 1 cup. Combine broccoli, chopped onion, parmesan cheese, mayonnaise and lemon juice. Spoon into centers of onion halves.

Melt butter. Blend in flour and salt. Add milk and cook until thick, stirring constantly. Remove from heat and blend in cream cheese. Spoon sauce over onion halves and bake uncovered in 375 degree oven for 20 minutes.

Stuffed Sweet Potatoes

6 servings.

6 medium-sized sweet potatoes
¼ cup butter, softened
1 tablespoon brown sugar
1 teaspoon salt
Dash pepper
Hot milk
⅔ cup miniature marshmallows
¼ cup chopped walnuts

Scrub the potatoes with a brush. Bake in 425 degree oven for 40 minutes or until done. Cut slice from top of each. Scoop out inside, being careful not to break shell. Mash potatoes with butter, brown sugar, salt, pepper and enough hot milk to moisten. Beat until fluffy. Fold in ⅓ cup tiny marshmallows and chopped walnuts.

Pile mixture lightly into the potato shells. Top with remaining tiny marshmallows. Bake in 350 degree oven for 15-20 minutes or until thoroughly hot and browned.

Dijon Au Gratin Potatoes

8 servings.

3½ pounds baking potatoes
Salt
Freshly ground pepper
¾ teaspoon dried thyme
10 ounces havarti cheese, shredded
1⅓ cups half and half
1⅓ cups chicken stock
¼ cup Dijon mustard

Peel potatoes and cut each into ⅛″ thick slices. Arrange ⅓ potatoes in overlapping slices in large oven-to-table dish coated with vegetable oil spray. Generously season potatoes with salt and pepper. Sprinkle with one-third of thyme and one-third of cheese. Top with 2 more layers potatoes, seasonings and cheese.

Whisk together half and half, chicken stock and Dijon mustard in bowl and pour mixture over potatoes. Bake in 400 degree oven 50-60 minutes, or until potatoes are tender when pierced with knife and top is golden and crusty. Serve warm.

Spinach or Broccoli Casserole

4 servings.

1 package frozen spinach or broccoli, thawed and drained
16 ounces low fat cottage cheese
¼ pound mild cheddar cheese, grated
3 eggs, slightly beaten
1 tablespoon margarine
1 tablespoon flour
Dash salt and pepper

Mix all ingredients together in a casserole dish. Bake for 1 hour-1 hour 30 minutes at 350 degrees. If desired, cook longer to form a crust on top.

Spinach Delight

8 servings.

3 12 ounce packages frozen
spinach souffle
1 medium onion,
peeled and thinly sliced
4 firm medium-sized tomatoes, diced

Partially thaw spinach souffles until they reach a mushy consistency. Preheat oven to 350 degrees. Arrange onion slices evenly on bottom of 9″ x 13″ baking dish. Cover with partially thawed spinach souffles. Arrange diced tomatoes on top of spinach and then top with grated cheese. Cover with aluminum foil and bake in preheated 350 degree oven for 1 hour.

Summer Squash Casserole

6 servings.

2 pounds crookneck squash,
(6 cups) sliced
¼ cup chopped onion
1 10.75 ounce can cream of
chicken soup
1 cup sour cream
1 cup shredded carrots
½ cup melted butter
1 8 ounce package herb stuffing

Cook squash and onion in boiling water for 5 minutes. Drain. Combine soup, sour cream and carrots. Fold in squash and onion. Add butter to stuffing. Spread one half of stuffing in bottom of 12″ x 7½″ pan or round casserole. Top with vegetable mixture. Sprinkle remaining stuffing over vegetables. Bake in 350 degree oven for 25-30 minutes.

Spicy Acorn Squash

4 servings.

2 small acorn squash
4 tablespoons fresh orange juice
Ground ginger
Ground nutmeg

Preheat oven to 375 degrees. Halve the squash from stem end to bottom. Remove seeds and discard. Slice a thin piece off the bottoms so that squash will stand straight. Arrange the 4 halves in a shallow baking pan just to fit. Place 1 tablespoon orange juice in each cavity. Sprinkle lightly with ginger and nutmeg. Cover the dish well with aluminum foil; bake for 1 hour - 1 hour 30 minutes, or until tender. Remove from oven, discard foil; let rest for 5 minutes before serving, so juice can penetrate squash.

§ *Calories: 98 Fat: .3gm Cholesterol: 0mg Sodium: 7mg*

Escalloped Tomatoes

4 to 6 servings.

1 28 ounce can peeled tomatoes, chopped
4 slices toast, cubed
1 tablespoon minced onions
¼ cup melted butter
1 cup cubed mozzarella cheese
1 cup cubed cheddar cheese
Salt and pepper

Mix together all ingredients in a 2 quart casserole. Bake uncovered at 375 degrees for 45 minutes.

Confetti Vegetable Ring

8 servings.

1 cup carrots, cooked and mashed
1 cup frozen, chopped broccoli
10 ounces frozen whole kernel corn
1 cup milk
1 cup cracker crumbs
½ cup sharp shredded cheddar cheese
¼ cup minced onion
⅓ cup butter or margarine, softened
Salt
Black pepper
⅛ teaspoon cayenne pepper
4 eggs

Combine carrots, broccoli, corn, milk, cracker crumbs, cheese, onion and butter in large mixing bowl. Season to taste with salt, pepper and cayenne pepper.

Beat eggs until frothy. Blend into carrot mixture lightly. Pour into greased 2 quart ring mold. Bake in 350 degree oven for 30-40 minutes or until knife inserted near center comes out clean.

Turn out onto warm platter and fill center with other hot cooked vegetables if desired.

Vegetable Medley

6 servings.

1 16 ounce package frozen broccoli, carrots and cauliflower combination, thawed and drained
1 10.75 can condensed cream of mushroom soup
1 cup (8 ounces) shredded Swiss cheese
⅓ cup sour cream
½ teaspoon black pepper
1 4 ounce jar chopped pimento, drained (optional)
1 2.8 ounce can French fried onions

Combine vegetables, soup, ½ cup cheese, sour cream, pepper, pimentos and half can French fried onions. Pour into 1 quart casserole. Bake covered in 350 degree oven for 30 minutes. Top with remaining cheese and onions. Bake uncovered for 5 minutes longer.

For Microwave:
Prepare as above, cook covered, on high for 8 minutes. Turn halfway through. Top with remaining cheese and onions. Cook, uncovered on high for 1 minute or until cheese melts.

Garden Vegetables with Cheese Sauce

8 servings.

1 **pound fresh broccoli**
1 **medium head cauliflower**
4-5 **carrots**
3 **tablespoons butter**
2 **tablespoons flour**
1 **teaspoon grated lemon peel**
½ **teaspoon salt**
Dash of pepper
¾ **cup milk**
1 **egg**
1 **cup sour cream**
¼ **cup grated parmesan cheese**
Cayenne pepper
Parsley

Steam vegetables and set aside. In saucepan melt butter, stir in flour, lemon peel, salt and pepper. Stir in milk. Cook, stirring continually, until bubbly. Pour some of sauce in a bowl with the beaten egg. Blend and pour egg mixture into sauce. Cook a few more minutes then stir in sour cream and parmesan cheese. Add a dash of cayenne pepper to taste.

Pour sauce over vegetables, using only enough to coat. Garnish with parsley.

J's Veggie Casserole

6 to 8 servings.

2 **fresh yellow crookneck squash**
2 **zucchini squash**
2 **fresh pattypan squash**
2 **fresh carrots**
½ **package cherry tomatoes**
1 **onion**
Sprigs of rosemary or thyme

Cut vegetables in large pieces. Place in casserole that has been coated with a non-stick vegetable spray. Season to taste. Place rosemary or thyme sprigs on top. Cover and bake in 350 degree oven just until tender, stirring once. Stir just before serving.

§ *Calories: 54 Fat: .5gm Cholesterol: 0mg Sodium: 17mg*

Baked Yams with
Sour Cream & Chives

6 servings.

2 pounds evenly sized and
shaped yams
2 teaspoons unsalted butter, softened
¼ cup sour cream
2 teaspoons chopped chives

Preheat oven to 400 degrees. Wash yams and rub lightly with butter. Place yams on baking sheet and bake 30 minutes. Prick skin of yams and return to oven for 30 minutes more or until tender. Remove pointed ends of yams and slice crosswise into 1½″ thick slices. Lay slices flat on plate and garnish each with 1 teaspoon sour cream and ¼ teaspoon chopped chives. Serve immediately.

Zucchini Florentine

6 servings.

6 small zucchini, cut in ¼″ slices
2 tablespoons butter
1 cup evaporated milk
1 teaspoon salt
¼ teaspoon pepper
3 eggs, slightly beaten
¼ teaspoon garlic salt
¼ teaspoon paprika

Place zucchini in 1½ quart casserole and add butter. Bake in 400 degree oven for 15 minutes. Combine remaining ingredients, except paprika, and pour over zucchini. Sprinkle with paprika. Set casserole in shallow pan, filling pan 1″ deep with hot water. Bake in 350 degree oven for 40 minutes or until knife inserted halfway between center and edge comes out clean.

New Orleans Zucchini

6 servings.

6 medium zucchini, sliced
1 onion, chopped
3 tablespoons butter
1 tablespoon flour
2 8 ounce cans tomatoes, chopped
1 green pepper, chopped
1 teaspoon salt
1 tablespoon brown sugar
1 bay leaf
4 whole cloves
Bread crumbs
Grated cheddar cheese

Boil zucchini in salted water for 3 minutes. Drain and set aside. Saute onion in butter. Add flour. Stir together in pan until blended. Add tomatoes, green pepper, and the zucchini, mixing well. Add salt, brown sugar, bay leaf and cloves and pour into a baking dish. Cover with bread crumbs and grated cheese. Bake uncovered in 350 degree oven for 30 minutes.

Zucchini Souffle

6 to 8 servings.

1½ pounds zucchini, cut in slices
2 tablespoons shredded onion
¼ cup chopped green pepper
1 teaspoon salt
2 tablespoons mayonnaise
½ cup grated cheddar cheese
3 eggs, separated
½ cup buttered crumbs

Place zucchini in a sauce pan with onion, green pepper, and salt. Add ½ cup boiling water, cover and cook until vegetables are tender. Remove lid and let cook until liquid is entirely evaporated. Vegetables should be quite dry. Mash thoroughly, using a potato masher or electric mixer. Add mayonnaise, cheese and beaten egg yolks. Fold in stiffly beaten egg whites, turn into greased casserole or baking dish. Sprinkle top with buttered crumbs and bake in 350 degree oven for 45 minutes, or until firm. Serve at once.

Curried Raisin Rice

10 servings.

1 medium onion, diced
3 tablespoons butter
2 cups long grain rice
2 teaspoons curry powder
4 cups water
½ cup raisins
2 teaspoons chicken bouillon or 2 cubes
¼ cup slivered almonds, toasted

Cook onion in butter until tender. Add rice, curry powder, water, raisins and chicken bouillon. Cover pan, steam rice until done without opening, about 15 minutes. Toast almonds in 350 degree oven for 5 minutes. Add toasted almonds just before serving.

Elegant Wild Rice

6 servings.

1 cup raw wild rice
5½ cups defatted chicken stock or water
1 cup shelled pecan halves
1 cup yellow raisins
Grated rind of 1 large orange
¼ cup chopped fresh mint
4 green onions, thinly sliced
¼ cup olive oil
⅓ cup fresh orange juice
1½ teaspoons salt
Freshly ground black pepper

Put rice in a strainer and run under cold water; rinse thoroughly. Place rice in a medium-size heavy saucepan. Add stock or water and bring to a rapid boil. Adjust heat to a gentle simmer and cook uncovered for 45 minutes. After 30 minutes check for doneness; rice should not be too soft. Place a thin towel inside a colander and turn rice into the colander and drain. Transfer drained rice to a bowl.

Add remaining ingredients to rice and toss gently. Adjust seasonings to taste. Let mixture stand for 2 hours to allow flavors to develop. Serve at room temperature.

Mixed Rice Pilaf

10 to 12 servings.

1½ cups wild and long grain rice
3 cups water
1½ teaspoons instant chicken bouillon
2 cups sliced fresh mushrooms
2 cups sliced celery
½ cup butter
1 pound artichoke hearts, chopped
½ cup sliced green onions
3 tablespoons chopped pimento
1½ teaspoons grated lemon peel
1½ teaspoons lemon juice
1 teaspoon salt
¾ teaspoon thyme
⅛ teaspoon pepper
Parsley

Combine rice, water and bouillon in three-quart saucepan. Bring to a boil. Cover and simmer for 30 minutes. Rice should be undercooked. Do not drain.

Cook mushrooms and celery in butter until tender. Stir in artichoke hearts, green onions, pimento, lemon peel, lemon juice, salt, thyme and pepper.

Stir mushroom mixture into rice. Turn into shallow 2 quart casserole dish. Cover and bake in 350 degree oven for 45-55 minutes.

Fresh Broccoli Pasta

3 to 4 servings.

8 ounces uncooked pasta
1-1½ cups cooked broccoli florets, drained (measure broccoli after cooking and press gently into cup)
5 medium or large fresh basil leaves
3 tablespoons butter
¾ cup whipping cream
1 cup grated parmesan cheese
Salt and pepper

Cook pasta according to package directions until tender; drain. In bowl of food processor fitted with steel blade, combine broccoli, basil leaves, butter and cream. Puree mixture. Add cheese and process until just blended. Mix into drained cooked pasta, stirring until coated. Cook, stirring, over moderate heat until heated through. Season with salt and pepper to taste.

Pasta Primavera

6 servings.

1 **pound uncooked corkscrew pasta**
¼ **cup chopped fresh basil**
2 **tablespoons mustard**
1 **tablespoon chopped garlic**
¼ **cup olive oil**
2 **tablespoons lemon juice**
¼ **cup shredded provolone cheese**
1 **tablespoon wine vinegar**
Salt and pepper
1½ **cups vegetables of your choice, chopped, slightly cooked**
¼ **cup grated parmesan cheese**

Cook pasta in boiling, salted water until cooked. Drain, rinse with cold water. Combine basil, mustard, garlic, oil, lemon juice, provolone cheese and vinegar in bowl. Add to pasta, toss to mix well. Let stand in refrigerator several hours or overnight. Season to taste with salt and pepper. Add vegetables and sprinkle with parmesan cheese.

Stuffed Shells in Sauce

6 to 8 servings.

1 **10 ounce package frozen spinach, cooked and drained**
1 **cup ricotta cheese**
½ **cup grated parmesan cheese**
½ **cup sour cream**
1.62 **ounce package vegetable soup mix**
1 **egg, beaten**
6 **ounces large shells for stuffing, cooked and drained**
1 **32 ounce jar spaghetti sauce**
Mozzarella cheese, shredded

Combine spinach with next 5 ingredients. Spoon mixture into each shell. Arrange stuffed shells in a 9" x 13" glass dish. Pour spaghetti sauce over all. Sprinkle cheese on top. Microwave on high power 10 minutes and then on medium power for 10 minutes.

Can be used as an appetizer if less sauce is used.

Pasta Fagioli

6 servings.

4 garlic cloves
1 tablespoon olive oil
1 tablespoon cooking oil
3 bay leaves
2 cups prepared spaghetti sauce
(fresh is preferred)
½ teaspoon salt (optional)
¼ teaspoon pepper
1½ quarts warm water
2 15 ounce cans chicken peas, drained
3 cups small pasta shells, cooked
Grated romano cheese

Brown garlic cloves in oils, add bay leaves, spaghetti sauce, salt and pepper. Simmer 10 minutes. Remove garlic cloves and bay leaves. Add warm water and drained peas. Simmer 10 minutes. Stir in cooked shells and heat for 20 minutes. Serve with romano cheese sprinkled on top.

Mixture can be prepared without shells and stored in the refrigerator or freezer. When ready to serve, cook and drain shells, reheat sauce, combine and simmer 20 minutes.

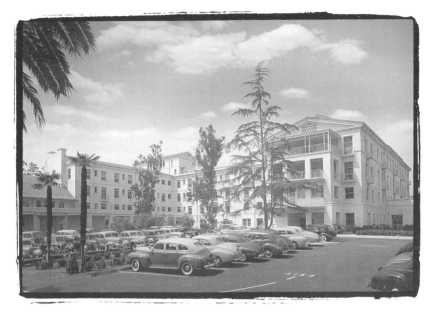

Collis P. and Howard Huntington Memorial Hospital, circa 1941

desserts

Almond Jumbles

Three cupfuls of soft sugar, two cupfuls of flour, half a cupful of butter, one teacupful

of loppered milk, five eggs well beaten, two tablespoonfuls of rose-water, three-quarters

of a pound of almonds, blanched and chopped very fine, one teaspoonful of soda dissolved.

Cream butter and sugar; stir in the beaten yolks, the milk, flour,

rose-water, almonds, and, lastly, the beaten whites very lightly and quickly;

drop in rings on buttered paper and bake at once.

The White House Cookbook © 1887

French Silk Pie

8 servings

1½ cups crushed vanilla wafers
1½ tablespoons sugar
6 tablespoons melted butter
½ pint whipping cream
¼ cup toasted almonds

Filling:
¾ cup butter at room temperature
1 cup plus 2 tablespoons sugar
1½ squares unsweetened chocolate, melted
1½ teaspoons vanilla extract
3 eggs

Combine the vanilla wafers, sugar and melted butter and press into a 9″ pie pan. Bake in 350 degree oven for 7 minutes. Remove from oven and cool. Pour filling into cooled pie shell and refrigerate. When ready to serve, top with whipped cream and almonds.

Filling:
Beat butter until creamy. Add sugar, a little at a time. Continue beating and add melted chocolate and vanilla. Add 2 eggs and beat 3 minutes. Add last egg and beat 3 minutes.

Lemon Chiffon Pie

8 servings.

1 6.75 ounce package lemon jello
¼ cup sugar
¼ cup hot water
1 6 ounce can frozen lemonade
1 13 ounce can evaporated milk
1 9″ pie shell, baked

Dissolve jello and sugar in hot water, cool until the consistency of syrup. Mix with lemonade. Pour evaporated milk into shallow tray, chill until crystals form. Whip milk until stiff. Fold in jello mixture. Pour into baked pie shell and chill.

Pineapple Mincemeat Pie

1 large pie.

Crust:
1 unbaked pie crust
½ cup flaked coconut

Topping:
⅔ cup sifted all-purpose flour
½ cup brown sugar, packed
1 teaspoon cinnamon
¼ teaspoon salt
¼ cup butter or margarine
2 tablespoons grated cheddar cheese

Filling:
1 15.25 ounce can pineapple tidbits
1 28 ounce jar prepared mincemeat
⅓ cup chopped macadamia or other nuts

Crust:
Place coconut in bottom of pie crust.

Topping:
Combine flour, brown sugar, cinnamon and salt. Cut in butter and cheese to form a crumb mixture.

Filling:
Drain and discard ¼ cup syrup from pineapple. Combine remaining pineapple and syrup with the mincemeat. Turn into coconut crust. Top with cheese crumb topping mixture. Sprinkle with nuts.

Bake below oven center in 425 degree oven for 15-20 minutes until crust begins to brown. Reduce heat to a moderate 350 degree oven and continue cooking 25-30 minutes longer. Cool.

Chocolate Angel Pie

6 to 8 servings.

Meringue Shell:
2 egg whites
¼ teaspoon cream of tartar
Pinch salt
½ cup sugar
½ teaspoon vanilla extract
3 tablespoons chopped pecans

Filling:
1 pint heavy cream
1 4 ounce sweet German chocolate bar
¼ cup hot water
Grated sweet chocolate
Chopped pecans

Meringue Shell:
In a bowl, beat egg whites until foamy; add cream of tartar and salt and beat until whites hold soft peaks. Beat in sugar, one tablespoon at a time and continue to beat until meringue holds very stiff peaks. Beat in vanilla and chopped nuts. Spoon the meringue into a well-buttered 9″ pie plate. With the back of a spoon, shape the sides of the shell by pushing meringue towards the edges and upwards. Bake in 275 degree oven for 1 hour. Turn off heat, leave oven door ajar and let meringue dry in the oven for 1 hour.

Filling:
Whip cream until stiff. Melt chocolate with hot water, mixing to dissolve (mixture should not become too hot). Let chocolate mixture cool slightly, then fold gently into whipped cream. Mound into cooled meringue shell and refrigerate for at least 30 minutes. Sprinkle grated chocolate and extra chopped pecans on top if desired.

Granny's Upside Down Apple Pie

1 pie.

⅓ cup unsalted butter,
softened but not melted
1½-1¾ cups large pecan halves
½ cup brown sugar, packed
Pastry for 2-crust 9″ deep dish pies
6 large Granny Smith apples, peeled
and thinly sliced (about 3¼ pounds)
1 tablespoon lemon juice
1 tablespoon flour
½ cup sugar
1 teaspoon ground cinnamon
1 teaspoon freshly ground nutmeg
Salt
2 tablespoons unsalted butter,
cut into small bits
Vanilla ice cream or Creme Fraiche

Spread softened butter evenly over bottom and sides of 9″ deep-dish pie pan. Arrange pecans, rounded side down, starting at center of pan bottom and working up to 1 row on sides, pressing them into butter. Sprinkle brown sugar evenly over pecans. Place pastry crust carefully over pecan mixture and gently press into place.

Toss apples in large bowl with lemon juice. Combine flour, sugar, cinnamon, nutmeg and salt. Add to apples and toss until combined. Place apple slices in pastry crust, mounding them in center. Dot surface with 2 tablespoons butter bits. Cover with other pastry crust. Fold top edge of crust over edge of bottom crust. Press gently to seal edges. Raise edge slightly up from edge of pan. Decoratively pierce or slash crust for steam to escape. Place pan on baking tray for easy handling.

Bake in center of oven at 400 degrees or until well browned, about 1 hour. (Test for doneness by piercing crust with point of small knife. If apples seem firm, bake pie longer, using foil to protect any very dark areas on crust.)

Remove from oven and let pie rest at room temperature 5 minutes. Invert onto serving plate. (As pie settles, outer crust may crack and have to be pressed back into shape). Serve warm or at room temperature with vanilla ice cream or Creme Fraiche.

Apple Zest

6 servings.

1 pie crust
3 large Granny Smith apples
½ cup sugar
1 teaspoon cinnamon

Topping:
½ cup apricot preserves
2 tablespoons butter or margarine
Water

Preheat oven to 400 degrees. Make pie crust and place in small rectangular baking dish. Pare, core and slice apples. Place in bowl with sugar and cinnamon. Mix well.

Arrange apples on pie crust in one overlapping layer. Bake in 400 degree oven for 15 minutes, lower temperature to 350 degrees and bake for another 15 minutes.

Topping:
Heat together the apricot preserves and butter until the butter is melted. Add just enough water to make mixture loose. Remove pan from oven and brush with topping mixture. Return to oven for 10 minutes. May be served warm or at room temperature.

Pecan Pie

8 servings.

½ cup sugar
1 tablespoon butter
½ cup white Karo syrup
Pinch of salt
1¼ cups pecans
3 eggs
1 teaspoon vanilla extract
1 9″ pie shell, unbaked
Whipped cream

Combine first 7 ingredients and pour into unbaked pie shell. Bake in 400 degree oven for 15 minutes. Reduce oven temperature to 350 degrees and continue to bake for 30-35 minutes or until knife inserted in center of pie comes out clean. Serve warm or cold. Top with whipped cream.

Upside Down Pumpkin Pie

10 to 12 servings.

1 29 ounce can pumpkin
1¼ cups sugar
2 teaspoons cinnamon
½ teaspoon ginger
1 12 ounce can evaporated milk
3 eggs, well beaten
1 teaspoon nutmeg
1 18.25 ounce package
yellow cake mix
1 cup chopped nuts
1 cup melted butter
Whipped cream

Combine first 7 ingredients. Mix and pour into a 9″ x 12″ baking dish. Sprinkle cake mix over mixture and then top with nuts. Drizzle butter over all. Bake in 350 degree oven for 1 hour. Cool and serve with whipped cream.

Peach Clafouti

8 servings.

Butter
4 tablespoons sugar
5 large peaches peeled and sliced
2 cups half and half or
1 cup heavy cream and
1 cup half and half
3 eggs
¼ cup flour
Pinch salt
¼ cup sugar
1 teaspoon vanilla extract

Heavily butter a 12″ diameter or 1½ quart baking dish. Sprinkle with 4 tablespoons sugar. Lay in the peaches. In a blender, combine the balance of the ingredients and blend. Pour over peaches. Bake at 375 degrees for 40-50 minutes, until puffed and golden.

Serve barely warm. If refrigerated, reheat at 170 degrees before serving.

John Miller's Grandmother's Persimmon Pudding

10 to 12 servings.

1 cup dates
1 cup dark rum
1 cup pulp from very ripe persimmons
1 cup sugar
1 egg, beaten
1¼ cups flour
1 teaspoon baking powder
1 teaspoon baking soda
½ teaspoon salt
½ teaspoon nutmeg
1 teaspoon cinnamon
½ cup milk
4 tablespoons butter, melted
1 teaspoon vanilla extract
1 cup chopped walnuts or pecans

Combine dates and rum, set aside. Beat persimmon pulp and gradually add sugar, beating continuously. Add egg and combine well. Sift dry ingredients together. Add alternately to persimmon mixture with milk. Add melted butter and vanilla. Mix in dates, rum and add chopped nuts. Pour batter into 2 buttered and floured 9″ x 5″ x 3″ pans, filling each three-quarters full. Bake in 325 degree oven for 1 hour.

Especially good when served warm with whipped cream.

Creme Brulee

6 servings.

1 quart cream (1 pint half and half and 1 pint whipping cream)
2 tablespoons sugar
8 egg yolks
2 teaspoons vanilla extract
Light brown sugar

Heat cream just to warm. Do not scald. Stir in sugar, slowly add 8 well beaten yolks. Add vanilla. Pour into 13″ x 9″ x 2″ baking dish and put in baine marie (dish of warm water). Bake in 325 degree oven until quite firm, approximately 40 minutes or more. Check with toothpick.

Cool and sprinkle with ¼″ of brown sugar on top and put under broiler to burn slightly. Watch carefully—only takes about 3 minutes.

Caramel Cheesecake Flan

12 servings.

¾ cup sugar
2 8 ounce packages cream cheese, softened
1 14 ounce can sweetened condensed milk
4 eggs
1½ teaspoons vanilla extract
½ teaspoon salt
1 cup water

Heat sugar in heavy skillet over medium heat, stirring constantly until melted and caramel colored. Pour into ungreased 9″ round cake pan, tilting to coat bottom evenly.

Beat cheese until fluffy. Gradually beat in milk until smooth. Add eggs, vanilla and salt and beat well. On low speed, gradually beat in water until smooth. Carefully pour into prepared pan. Set pan in larger pan and fill outer pan with hot water to come 1″ up side of pan. Bake in 350 degree oven for 55 minutes-1 hour or until top springs back when lightly touched.

Cool, then chill thoroughly. Loosen side of flan with knife. Invert onto serving plate with rim. Garnish as desired.

English Toffee Torte

12 servings.

16 egg whites, room temperature
½ teaspoon cream of tartar
Dash salt
2 cups sugar
4 cups heavy cream
8 Skor candy bars, crushed

To egg whites, add cream of tartar and salt. Beat egg whites, adding sugar gradually until stiff peaks form. Line cookie sheets with foil with an 8″ circle drawn in center and shape meringues in 3 circles.

Bake in 275 degree oven for 1 hour. Turn oven off but do not remove for 2 hours.

Whip cream until stiff and fold in crushed candy bars. Arrange in layers, beginning with meringue and alternating between filling and meringue. Chill at least 24 hours.

Chocolate Peppermint Torte

12 servings.

1 cup chocolate wafer crumbs
2 tablespoons butter, melted
½ cup butter, softened
¾ cup sugar
3 ounces unsweetened chocolate, melted
1 teaspoon vanilla extract
¾ teaspoon peppermint extract
3 eggs
½ cup cream, whipped
1 ounce unsweetened chocolate, grated

Prepare crust by combining the chocolate wafer crumbs and melted butter. Lightly press into bottom of a 9″ cake pan with removable bottom. Bake in 350 degree oven for 7 minutes or until toasted. Cool.

In a mixer bowl, beat butter until creamy; gradually add sugar and beat until light and fluffy. Then beat in chocolate, vanilla, and peppermint. Add eggs, one at a time, beating for 3 minutes after each addition. Fold in the whipped cream, then spoon into the crumb crust. Sprinkle with the grated chocolate.

Cover lightly and chill at least 4 hours or overnight.

Black Russian Cake

10 to 12 servings.

¼ cup Kahlua
¼ cup vodka
1 18.25 ounce package yellow cake mix
1 small package instant chocolate fudge pudding mix
4 eggs
1 cup oil
¾ cup water
Powdered sugar

Combine all ingredients, mix for 2 minutes at medium speed. Bake in an angel food tube pan at 350 degrees for 45-50 minutes. Cool. Sift powdered sugar over cake.

Amber Rum Cake

1 cake.

1 18.25 ounce yellow cake mix
1 3 ounce package lemon instant pudding and pie filling mix
4 eggs
1 cup apricot nectar
1 cup dark rum
¼ cup oil
¼ cup currants or raisins
½ cup water
1 cup sugar

Preheat oven to 350 degrees. Grease and flour a 12 cup bundt or 10″ tube pan. Combine cake mix, pudding mix, eggs, ½ cup nectar, ½ cup rum, oil and currants in large bowl. Blend well. Then beat at medium speed for 2 minutes. Turn into pan and bake for 45 minutes or until done.

In a small sauce pan, mix and bring to boil the water, ½ cup nectar, ½ cup rum and the sugar. Let cake stand 10 minutes. Turn onto plate and drizzle syrup mixture over cake.

Cinnamon-Apple Cake

6 servings.

½ cup butter or margarine
1 cup sugar
1 egg
1 cup flour
½ teaspoon baking powder
½ teaspoon baking soda
½ teaspoon cinnamon
3 medium apples, pared, diced

Cream butter and sugar together. Add egg and beat well. Combine flour with baking powder, soda and cinnamon and add to above mixture. Stir in apples. Pour into ungreased 8″ x 8″ square baking pan and bake in 350 degree oven for 45 minutes.

Soused Apple Cake

10 servings.

½ cup brandy
4 cups coarsely chopped apples
2 cups sugar
½ cup salad oil
2 eggs
2 cups flour
2 teaspoons cinnamon
2 teaspoons baking soda
1 teaspoon nutmeg
1 teaspoon salt
¼ teaspoon ground cloves
1 cup chopped walnuts
1 cup plumped raisins

Lemon Cheese Icing:
1 3 ounce package cream cheese
2 tablespoons half and half
½ cup soft butter
4 cups sifted powdered sugar
1 tablespoon lemon juice
2 teaspoons grated lemon peel
1 teaspoon vanilla extract
Dash salt

Pour brandy over apples. Set aside. Beat together the sugar, oil, eggs. Sift together all dry ingredients and add this to sugar mixture; add apples, walnuts and raisins. Pour into oiled 9″ x 13″ pan. Bake in 325 oven for 1 hour. Serve warm or cold with whipped cream or Lemon Cheese Icing.

Lemon Cheese Icing:
Soften cream cheese to room temperature. Add half and half, butter, sugar, lemon juice, lemon peel, vanilla and salt. Beat until fluffy. Tint pale yellow if you wish with yellow food coloring. Add more sugar or cream if necessary to spread.

Chocolate Chip
Sour Cream Walnut Cake

16 to 20 servings.

½ cup butter or margarine
1 cup sugar
3 eggs, separated
3 tablespoons grated lemon peel
2 cups sifted flour
1 teaspoon baking soda
1 teaspoon baking powder
¼ teaspoon salt
1 cup sour cream
1 cup semi-sweet chocolate chips
1 cup chopped walnuts

Sauce:
½ cup sugar
2 tablespoons orange juice
2 tablespoons lemon juice

Cream butter and sugar. Beat in egg yolks, one at a time. Add lemon peel. Sift flour with baking soda, baking powder and salt. Add to creamed mixture, alternately with sour cream. Beat egg whites and fold into cake batter with chocolate chips and nuts. Turn into greased and floured tube pan. Bake at 350 degrees for 50 minutes or until done. While hot, baste with sauce.

Sauce:
Combine all ingredients and mix. Bring to a boil. Continue to boil, stirring constantly, until sugar has completely dissolved.

Orange Chocolate Bit Cake

16 servings.

1 cup sugar
1¾ cups cake flour
1 cup orange juice
3 eggs
¼ teaspoon salt
1 cup vegetable oil
1 cup chocolate chips

Blend all ingredients together and pour into well greased bundt pan. Bake in preheated 350 degree oven for 45-50 minutes.

Citrus Sunshine Cake

1 cake.

⅔ cup margarine, softened
1 tablespoon grated orange peel
1½ teaspoons grated lemon peel
1½ cups sugar
3 eggs
2½ cups sifted cake flour
2½ teaspoons baking powder
¾ teaspoon salt
2 tablespoons lemon juice
¼ cup orange juice
½ cup milk

Frosting:
½ cup margarine, softened
2 teaspoons grated orange peel
1 pound powdered sugar
2 tablespoons orange juice

Combine margarine, orange peel and lemon peel; mix well. Add sugar gradually; cream until light and fluffy. Add eggs, one at a time; beat well after each. Sift together flour, baking powder and salt; add to creamed mixture alternately with lemon juice, orange juice and milk; a small amount at a time. Beat after each addition until smooth. Bake in 2 wax paper-lined 9" x 1½" round cake pans in a 375 degree oven for 25-30 minutes. Cool. Remove from pans and remove paper liner from bottom of cake.

Frosting:
Combine margarine and orange peel in bowl. Add powdered sugar and orange juice. Beat until spreading consistency. Spread on cooled cake.

Cherry Delight Cake

12 to 15 servings.

2 21 ounce cans cherry pie filling
1 18.25 ounce package cake mix
(white, yellow or chocolate)
1 cup slivered almonds
¾ cup melted margarine or butter
Whipped cream

Spread pie filling in 9" x 13" pan. Sprinkle dry cake mix over filling. Top with nuts. Pour melted butter evenly over the mix. Bake in 350 degree oven for 1 hour until nuts brown. Serve at room temperature topped with whipped cream, if desired.

The Very Best Carrot Cake

12 to 16 servings.

2 cups flour
2 teaspoons baking soda
2 teaspoons cinnamon
½ teaspoon salt
3 eggs
1¾ cups sugar
¾ cup vegetable oil
¾ cup buttermilk
2 teaspoons vanilla extract
1 8.25 ounce can crushed unsweetened, pineapple, drained
2 cups shredded carrots
1 cup chopped walnuts
1 3.5 ounce can flaked coconut (optional)

Buttermilk Frosting:
¾ cups sugar
½ cup buttermilk
½ cup butter
1 tablespoon white corn syrup
½ teaspoon soda
1 teaspoon vanilla extract

In medium bowl, sift together flour, soda, cinnamon and salt. Stir to blend. In large bowl, beat eggs and slowly blend in sugar. Add oil, buttermilk and vanilla and stir well. Stir in flour mixture until blended. Stir in pineapple, carrots, nuts and coconut. Pour into lightly greased and floured 9″ x 13″ baking pan. Bake at 350 degrees for 55-60 minutes (325 degrees for glass pan) or until cake tests done in center. Pierce cake all over with a fork. Pour buttermilk frosting over hot cake. Let stand until cool. Cut into serving pieces.

Buttermilk Frosting:
Combine sugar, buttermilk, butter, corn syrup and soda in saucepan. Bring to boil and continue to boil for five minutes. Remove from heat and stir in vanilla. Pour over hot cake.

Pumpkin Cake

8 to 10 servings.

4 eggs
2 cups all-purpose flour
2 teaspoons baking soda
½ teaspoon salt
1 teaspoon ground cloves
2 teaspoons ground cinnamon
¼-½ teaspoon powdered ginger
2 teaspoons nutmeg
2 cups sugar
1 cup salad oil
1 16 ounce can pumpkin

Cream Cheese Frosting:
2 3 ounce packages cream cheese, softened
1 tablespoon rum extract or
1 teaspoon vanilla extract
1½ cups powdered sugar

Crack eggs into a large mixing bowl and let warm to room temperature, approximately 30 minutes. Preheat oven to 350 degrees. Sift flour with baking soda, salt, cloves, cinnamon, ginger and nutmeg. Set aside.

At high speed, beat eggs with sugar until light and fluffy. Beat in oil and pumpkin to blend well. At low speed, blend in flour mixture just until combined. Pour into ungreased 9″ tube pan. Bake for 55 minutes-1 hour.

Cool cake completely in pan. Remove from pan, place on plate and frost with cream cheese frosting.

Cream Cheese Frosting:
In medium bowl, combine cream cheese, rum extract and powdered sugar. Mix on medium speed with electric mixer until creamy.

No Bake Fruit Cake

1 loaf.

1 pint whipping cream or Cool Whip
1 pound miniature marshmallows
1 pound whole walnuts
1 pound whole pecans
1 pound candied pineapple,
cut in small pieces
1 pound candied whole cherries
1 pound dates cut in half
2 pounds graham crackers, crushed

Mix whipping cream or Cool Whip and marshmallows. Set bowl in refrigerator for 2 days. Do not stir.

After 2 days, mix nuts and fruits together in a large bowl. Add graham crackers and mix well. Pour the whipping cream, marshmallow mixture into the nuts and fruit mixture. Mix well again.

Using enough wax paper to completely cover the cake, pour mixture on the wax paper and shape to the size of the bread loaf pan. Put in the loaf pan and place in refrigerator for 6 days before cutting.

By the sixth day, it should be firm enough to slice. There is no baking-just refrigeration.

Poppy Seed Cake

3 servings.

1 18.25 ounce package lemon cake mix
1 3.5 ounce package instant lemon
pudding mix
4 eggs
½ cup poppy seeds
1 cup hot water
½ cup vegetable oil
Powdered sugar

Combine first 6 ingredients and mix for 7 minutes. Pour cake into a greased bundt pan. Bake in 350 degree oven for 45-50 minutes. Once cake is cooled, remove from bundt pan and sprinkle with powdered sugar.

Cassata Cake

8 to 10 servings.

1 **pound ricotta cheese**
¼ **cup powdered sugar**
(can substitute 3 tablespoons honey)
½ **cup grated semi-sweet chocolate**
½ **cup chopped candied fruit or**
dried fruit
½ **cup chopped almonds**
3 **tablespoons rum or brandy**
1 **loaf shape pound cake,**
sliced lengthwise into 3-4 layers

Frosting:
2 **6 ounce packages chocolate chips**
¾ **cup strong coffee**
1 **cup cold butter**
(do not use margarine)

Beat the ricotta cheese until smooth. Mix with powdered sugar, semi-sweet chocolate, candied fruit, almonds and rum. To assemble, start with bottom layer of cake, top with filling. Continue to alternate a cake layer and filling, ending with a top layer of cake. Spread top and sides with frosting. Cover cake loosely and refrigerate overnight.

Frosting:
Combine chocolate and coffee in top of double boiler. Stir and melt. Beat until well blended. Remove from heat and beat in chunks of butter a little at a time until smooth. Chill in freezer or refrigerator until of spreading consistency.

Fantastic Chocolate Potato Cake

16 servings.

1 cup butter
2 cups sugar
2 cups flour, sifted
½ cup ground chocolate
½ cup chopped walnuts
2 teaspoons baking powder
1 teaspoon cinnamon
1 teaspoon ground cloves
4 eggs, separated
½ cup milk
1 cup hot mashed potatoes

Cream butter and sugar. Add to dry ingredients. Separate eggs. Stir yolk and add to dry ingredients. Beat whites stiff. Set aside. Add milk and hot potatoes. Stir in stiff beaten egg white. Beat entire mixture about 4 minutes on medium speed. Bake for 1 hour in 350 degree oven in greased angel food pan.

Serve plain or frosted with whipped cream.

Cranberry Cakeletts

6 servings.

¾ cup flour
½ teaspoon baking powder
½ teaspoon salt
2 cups fresh cranberries
1 cup chopped dates
3½ cups chopped walnuts
2 eggs
¾ cup sugar
1 teaspoon lemon extract

Sift together flour, baking powder and salt. Combine cranberries, dates and walnuts with flour mixture in large bowl. Toss fruit to evenly coat with flour mixture. Beat eggs, sugar and lemon extract together until light and fluffy. Pour over flour and fruit mixing thoroughly.

Line 2½" muffin pans with fluted paper baking cups, and pack fruit mixture into cups filling about two-thirds full. Bake in 300 degree oven for 45-50 minutes. Cool in pans for 15 minutes. Keeps in refrigerator for 2-3 weeks wrapped.

Black-Bottom Cupcakes

40 cupcakes.

1½ cups flour
1 cup sugar
1 teaspoon baking soda
⅓ cup oil
¼ cup cocoa
1 cup water
1 tablespoon vinegar
1 8 ounce package cream cheese
1 egg
⅓ cup sugar
1 6 ounce package chocolate chips

Combine first 7 ingredients. Fill paper-lined muffin cups one-third full of batter. Make filling by combining cream cheese with egg and sugar. Beat well and stir in chocolate chips. Put 1 tablespoon of filling on top of batter in each of the muffin cups. Bake in 350 degree oven for 15 minutes.

Streusel Topping Cupcakes

12 cupcakes.

2 cups Bisquick baking mix
2 tablespoons sugar
1 egg
⅔ cup water or milk

Topping:
⅓ cup Bisquick baking mix
⅓ cup brown sugar
⅓ teaspoon cinnamon
2 tablespoons firm margarine or butter

Heat oven to 400 degrees. Mix all ingredients except for topping. Beat well for about 30 seconds. Divide batter into 12 muffin cups lined with paper baking cups; sprinkle with topping. Bake for about 15 minutes.

Topping:
Combine Bisquick baking mix, brown sugar, cinnamon and margarine until crumbly. Spoon over cupcakes and bake as directed.

Cocoa-Cottage Cheese Cake

10 to 12 servings.

1 cup butter or margarine
1 cup sugar
1 cup brown sugar
2 eggs
¾ cup small curd cottage cheese
1 teaspoon vanilla extract
2 ⅔ cups cake flour
¼ cup cocoa
1 teaspoon salt
1 teaspoon baking soda
½ teaspoon baking powder
1¼ cups buttermilk
1 cup chopped nuts

Cream butter and sugars together. Add eggs, cottage cheese and vanilla extract. Beat well. Sift dry ingredients together and add alternately with buttermilk. Fold in nuts. Pour into a well-greased and lightly-floured 13″ x 9″ x 2″ oblong baking pan. Bake in 350 degree oven for 45-50 minutes. Top with your favorite frosting.

Deluxe Cheesecake

12 servings.

1 12 ounce box vanilla wafers
6 tablespoons butter, melted
5 eggs, separated
1 cup sugar
16 ounces cream cheese
16 ounces sour cream
1 teaspoon vanilla extract
1 tablespoon lemon juice

To make crumb crust, blend together vanilla wafers that have been crushed with melted butter. Press into bottom and sides of 9″ spring form pan. Beat 5 egg whites until stiff and set aside. Blend 5 egg yolks with remaining ingredients. Then fold in egg whites. Pour into crumb crust. Bake 1 hour in 325 degree oven. Do not open oven. Turn oven off and leave in for 1 more hour. Remove from oven, cool and then refrigerate.

Irish Chocolate Chip Cheesecake

12 servings.

2 cups graham cracker crumbs
¼ cup sugar
6 tablespoons butter, melted
2¼ pounds cream cheese, room temperature
1⅔ cups sugar
5 eggs, room temperature
1 cup Baileys Original Irish Cream
1 tablespoon vanilla extract
1 cup semi-sweet chocolate chips
1 cup chilled whipping cream
2 tablespoons sugar
1 teaspoon instant coffee powder
1 cup chocolate curls

For crust, preheat oven to 325 degrees. Coat 9″ diameter spring form pan with nonstick vegetable spray. Combine crumbs and sugar in pan. Stir in butter. Press mixture into bottom and 1″ up sides of pan. Bake until light brown, about 7 minutes. Maintain oven temperature at 325 degrees.

Using electric mixer, beat cream cheese until smooth. Gradually mix in sugar. Beat in eggs, 1 at a time. Blend in Baileys and vanilla. Sprinkle half of chocolate chips over crust. Spoon in filling. Sprinkle with remaining chocolate chips. Bake cake until puffed, springy in center and golden brown, about 1 hour 20 minutes. Cool cake completely.

Beat whipping cream, sugar and coffee powder until peaks form. Spread mixture over cooled cake. Garnish with chocolate curls. Cut into thin slices to serve.

Praline Cheesecake

18 servings.

1 18.25 ounce package German
chocolate cake mix with pudding
½ cup flaked coconut
⅓ cup margarine or butter, softened
1 egg
2 8 ounce packages cream cheese,
softened
2 eggs
¾ cup sugar
2 teaspoons vanilla extract
2 cups dairy sour cream
¼ cup brown sugar, packed
1 tablespoon vanilla extract
⅓ cup flaked coconut
⅓ cup chopped pecans

Heat oven to 350 degrees. Beat cake mix, ½ cup coconut, margarine and 1 egg in large bowl on low speed until crumbly. Press lightly in ungreased rectangular baking pan, 13" x 9" x 2".

Beat cream cheese, 2 eggs, sugar and 2 teaspoons vanilla until smooth and fluffy. Spread over cake mixture. Bake until set, about 25 minutes. Cool.

Mix sour cream, brown sugar and 1 tablespoon vanilla until smooth. Spread over cheesecake. Mix ⅓ cup coconut and the pecans; sprinkle over cheesecake. Cover and refrigerate at least 8 hours. Cut into diamond shapes to serve.

No Mess-No Fuss Cheesecake

12 servings.

1½ cups graham crackers, finely ground
¼ cup sugar
½ cup melted butter
1 pound cream cheese
1 pound cottage cheese
1½ cups sugar
4 eggs
Juice of ½ lemon, fresh
1 teaspoon vanilla extract
3 tablespoons flour
3 tablespoons cornstarch
½ pound butter, melted
1 pint sour cream

Combine first 3 ingredients to make graham cracker crust. Place in bottom of spring form pan and bake in 375 degree oven for 8 minutes.

Mix cream cheese, cottage cheese, sugar, eggs, lemon juice, vanilla, flour, cornstarch and melted butter in a food processor. Fold in sour cream. Pour over baked crust. Bake in 325 degree oven for 1 hour. Leave in oven for 2 hours with door open and heat off. Cool 6-12 hours in refrigerator before serving.

Pears Poached in Rum Raspberry Sauce

6 servings.

6 small fresh pears
1 package frozen red raspberries with sugar, thawed
2 tablespoons rum
⅓ cup whipped cream (optional)

Peel pears leaving fruit whole with stems intact. Place upright in crockpot. Blend raspberries in a blender until smooth. Add rum and pour over pears. Cook on low for 4-6 hours or until pears are tender. Chill. Serve with whipped cream if desired.

§ *Calories: 180 Fat: 3.2gm Cholesterol: 9mg Sodium: 3mg*

Pears in Red Wine

4 servings.

1 cup sugar
2 cups red wine
1 piece cinnamon stick (1½″ long)
4 whole allspice berries
Pinch freshly grated nutmeg
1 cardamom pod, crushed
2 whole cloves
2 Bosc pears, peeled, cored and halved

Combine all ingredients except pears in an 8 cup glass measure. Cook uncovered in microwave on high (100%) for 3 minutes. Stir well. Cover tightly with microwave plastic wrap. Cook at 100% for 5 minutes longer. Remove from oven. Arrange pears in an 8½″ x 7″ x 2½″ dish, cored side up, alternating wide and narrow ends. Pour liquid over pears. Cover tightly with microwave wrap and cook at 100% for 12 minutes.

Remove from oven and pierce plastic with the tip of a sharp knife. Cool pears in syrup. Serve pears with a little of the syrup. Other fruits such as peaches may be used.

Perfect Pear Crisp with Cardamom

4 to 6 servings.

1½ pounds pears, sliced
Grated zest of ½ lemon
¼ cup whole wheat flour
½ cup all-purpose flour
⅜ cup sugar
⅛ teaspoon salt
½ teaspoon ground cardamom
⅜ cup unsalted butter, diced
Whipped cream or vanilla ice cream

Mix sliced pears with grated lemon zest and place in 9″ pie dish. Combine whole wheat and all-purpose flours with sugar, salt and cardamom in bowl. Cut in butter with knives or pastry blender until mixture resembles coarse cornmeal. Distribute flour mixture over pears. Bake in 375 degree oven until pears are tender, topping is lightly browned and juices are building up around edges, about 40 minutes.

Serve plain or with whipped cream or vanilla ice cream.

Apple Crisp

8 servings.

6 large apples, peeled and sliced
2 tablespoons lemon juice
¼ cup water
½ teaspoon cinnamon
1 cup sugar
¾ cup flour
Pinch of salt
6 tablespoons margarine

Place apples in deep 2 quart casserole. Add lemon juice and water. Mix cinnamon with ½ cup sugar and sprinkle over the apples. Combine remaining sugar with the flour and salt. Work in margarine with finger tips until mixture resembles coarse cornmeal. Sprinkle over apples and pat with back of a spoon. Bake in 375 degree oven for 40-50 minutes or until apples are tender and crust is crisp.

Kiwi Fruit Sorbet

8 servings.

1 cup sugar
1½ cups water
8 kiwi fruit (3 ounces each), peeled
½ cup lime juice
Fresh strawberries

Combine sugar and water in saucepan. Bring to boil over high heat; boil 5 minutes and cool. Puree enough kiwi pulp in food processor to equal 2 cups puree. Add sugar syrup and lime juice to pulp. Pour into a 9″ square baking pan. Freeze until hardened. Turn frozen mixture into mixer bowl and beat until smooth, light and airy. Return to freezer.

To serve, scoop into dishes and surround with fresh strawberries.

Ice Cream Supra

12 servings.

4 ounces slivered almonds
¼ pound butter
1 cup brown sugar
1 cup shredded coconut
2½ cups crushed Rice Chex cereal
½ gallon vanilla ice cream
(brick-style), softened

Saute almonds in butter. In a bowl, mix brown sugar, shredded coconut and Rice Chex. Add sauteed almonds. Mix thoroughly. Put half of mixture in a 9″ x 13″ pan. Smooth ice cream over mixture. Add remaining cereal mixture. Smooth top and freeze.

Cranberry Apple Tart

10 to 12 servings.

Crust:
2 cups flour
⅛ teaspoon salt
6 tablespoons butter
¼ cup shortening, chilled
4-5 tablespoons ice water

Filling:
1¼ cups apple juice
1¾ cups sugar
4 large Golden Delicious apples,
peeled, cored and cut into ½″ cubes
12 ounces cranberries

Pecan Streusel Topping:
½ cup finely chopped pecans
½ cup flour
⅓ cup brown sugar, firmly packed
6 tablespoons butter, melted
Whipped cream

Crust:
Combine flour and salt in bowl. Cut in butter and shortening until coarse meal forms. Mix in enough water to form ball. Wrap dough and refrigerate at least 1 hour.

Roll dough out to ⅛″ round and place in 10″ tart pan with removable sides. Trim and finish edges. Refrigerate 30 minutes. Preheat oven to 400 degrees and pierce crust lightly with fork and fill with dried beans or pie weights. Bake 15 minutes. Remove beans and continue to bake 10 minutes. Cool to room temperature on rack. Reduce oven to 375 degrees.

Filling:
Heat apple juice and sugar over low heat stirring until sugar dissolves. Increase heat and bring to boil. Reduce heat and simmer 2 minutes. Stir in apples and cranberries. Return to boil. Reduce

heat and simmer until cranberries burst and apples are tender, stirring frequently, 8-10 minutes. Transfer to bowl and cool. Wrap tightly and refrigerate overnight. Bring to room temperature before transferring to tart pan.

Pecan Streusel Topping:
Mix all ingredients in large bowl until blended and crumbly.

To assemble, place baking sheet in oven on center rack and heat 5 minutes. Spoon filling into crust and sprinkle streusel topping evenly over filling. Place tart on hot baking sheet and cook until top is brown and filling bubbles, 30-35 minutes. Cool on rack. Serve with whipped cream.

Pumpkin & Pear Tart

16 servings.

Crust:
1¾ cups flour
¼ cup sugar
¼ teaspoon salt
1½ sticks butter
2 egg yolks beaten
⅓ cup finely chopped
crystallized ginger
1 teaspoon vanilla extract
4-5 tablespoons cold water

Filling:
2 large eggs
1 cup sugar
1 16 ounce can pumpkin
¼ cup whipping cream
¾ teaspoon ginger
¾ teaspoon coriander
½ teaspoon nutmeg
¼ teaspoon salt
½ stick butter

Topping:
2 pears, peeled, halved and cored
1 lemon, halved
2 teaspoons sugar
½ teaspoon cinnamon

Glaze:
¼ cup apricot jam
2 tablespoons brandy

Crust:
Combine flour, sugar and salt in large bowl. Cut in butter with pastry blender until mixture resembles coarse meal. Mix in egg yolks, ginger and vanilla. Stir in enough water to bind dough. Wrap in plastic and refrigerate for 15 minutes. Lightly butter a 10″ x 2″ spring form pan. Pat dough in pan and place in refrigerator for 30 minutes. Preheat oven to 375 degrees and bake crust for 10 minutes using pie weights and foil. Remove foil and bake 10 minutes. Cool crust.

Filling:
Beat eggs and 1 cup sugar to blend. Whisk in pumpkin, cream, ginger, coriander, nutmeg and salt. Melt butter in saucepan over medium-high heat. Stir butter until light brown. Whisk into pumpkin mixture. Pour into prepared crust.

Topping:
Slice pears lengthwise into ¼″ thick slices. Squeeze lemon over pears to prevent discoloration. Place pear slices on top of filling in a spoke-like design. Sprinkle with sugar and cinnamon. Bake tart until center no longer moves, about 1 hour 15 minutes. Cool on rack for 10 minutes.

Glaze:
Combine jam and brandy in saucepan. Cook over medium heat until jam is melted and smooth, stirring constantly. Brush pears gently with glaze.

Shredded Wheat Dessert (Poor Man's Baklava)

10 to 12 servings.

2 cups sugar
1 cup water
½ teaspoon lemon juice
1 10 ounce box shredded wheat (regular size)
2 cups milk, cold
16 ounces chopped nuts
1 tablespoon cinnamon
1 teaspoon sugar
¼ pound butter
½ cup whipped cream

Make syrup by boiling the sugar and water for 10 minutes. Add lemon juice, stir and set aside to cool. Dip each roll of shredded wheat lightly into the cold milk, one by one, put them on a towel to drain.

Combine the nuts, cinnamon and sugar. Open the centers of the rolls with a spoon and fill with the nut mixture. Place in a buttered pan, place a pat of butter on each roll or pour a spoonful of melted butter over each. Bake in 350 degree oven for 35-40 minutes. When baked, remove from oven and pour the cooled syrup over the rolls. Cover and let stand until cool. Serve with whipped cream.

Grand Marnier Fudge Sauce

1 cup.

3 squares unsweetened chocolate
¼ cup butter
1 cup powdered sugar
6 tablespoons heavy cream
1 teaspoon vanilla extract
1-2 tablespoons Grand Marnier

Over low heat melt chocolate and butter, stirring constantly with whisk. When melted, beat in sugar, add 3 tablespoons cream and continue to whisk. When well blended, whisk in remaining cream, vanilla and Grand Marnier.

Berry Fast Mousse

6 servings.

1½ cups fresh strawberries or
8 ounces frozen unsweetened whole
strawberries, thawed
1 8 ounce package cream cheese,
cut into small cubes
½ cup sifted powdered sugar
1 4 ounce container frozen whipped
dessert topping, thawed
Sliced fresh strawberries or
sliced almonds

In a blender container or food processor bowl combine strawberries, cream cheese and powdered sugar. Cover and blend or process until mixture is smooth, stopping and scraping sides as necessary. Pour into a mixing bowl. Fold in dessert topping.

Spoon mixture into 6 dessert dishes. Chill 3-4 hours or overnight. To serve, top with sliced strawberries or sprinkle with almonds.

Chocolate Mousse

4 servings.

1 cup heavy cream
3 teaspoons sugar
6 ounces semi-sweet chocolate chips
⅓ cup hot strong coffee
2 eggs
1 tablespoon rum or orange liqueur
Whipped cream
Chocolate shavings

In a food processor fitted with steel blade or in a blender, whip the cream and add sugar. Place whipped cream in bowl and wash the processor or blender parts.

Blend chocolate chips, add the strong coffee and process, until the chocolate is melted. Add the eggs and rum or liqueur and blend until smooth. Fold chocolate mixture into cream.

Transfer the mousse to dessert glasses and chill for at least 30 minutes or until firm. Garnish with whipped cream or chocolate shavings.

Chilled Grand Marnier Souffle

8 servings.

3 eggs, separated
½ cup sugar
3 ounces Grand Marnier
1 cup whipping cream
1 teaspoon vanilla extract
1 envelope unflavored gelatin
¼ cup cold water
1 12 ounce package frozen raspberries
¼ cup powdered sugar

In large mixing bowl, beat egg yolks until lemon colored. Add sugar and continue beating until creamy. Add 2 ounces Grand Marnier; set aside. In large bowl, beat egg whites until stiff but not dry; set aside. In third bowl, beat cream until stiff enough to stand in peaks; add vanilla and set aside.

Soften gelatin in cold water for 5 minutes, then stir over hot water until gelatin is dissolved; cool slightly. Stir dissolved gelatin mixture into egg mixture and combine thoroughly. Gently fold in beaten egg whites and whipped cream. Pour into souffle dish and chill several hours or overnight.

Thaw package of raspberries for 15 minutes. Place all berries, including juice, into a blender. Add powdered sugar and 1 ounce Grand Marnier. Blend until a smooth and thick sauce. Chill.

To serve, place a portion of souffle in individual dessert bowls and top with raspberry sauce.

Dee's Angel Fluff

12 servings.

¼ pound butter, softened
1½ cups powdered sugar
3 egg yolks
3 soft egg whites, stiffly beaten
1 pint whipping cream
Angel food cake, baked or purchased
1 5.7 ounce can flaked coconut

Cream butter and sugar. Add egg yolks one at a time, beating after each addition. Add lemon juice. Fold in egg whites and half of whipping cream.

Thinly slice angel food cake. Line 9″ x 13″ pan with half of cake slices. Pour half of the filling over slices. Layer balance of cake slices and cover rest with filling. Cover with reserved whipped cream. Top with flaked coconut. Refrigerate.

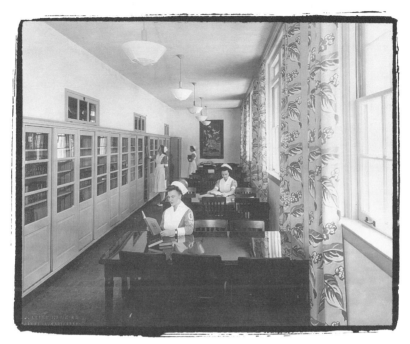

Library at nursing school of Huntington Memorial Hospital

candy and cookies

Hoarhound Candy

Boil two ounces of dried hoarhound in a pint and a half of water for about half an hour; strain and add three and a half pounds of brown sugar; boil over a hot fire until sufficiently hard; pour out in flat, well greased tins and mark sticks or small squares with a knife as soon as cool enough to retain its shape.

The White House Cookbook ©1887

Chocolate Surprise

2½ dozen.

1 12 ounce package chocolate chips
1 12 ounce package butterscotch chips
1 can Chinese noodles
1 cup chopped nuts (optional)

Melt both packages of chips in top of a large double boiler until smooth. Mix in Chinese noodles and nuts until thoroughly coated. Drop by teaspoons on cookie sheet, place in refrigerator until cooled, approximately 20 minutes. Serve immediately or store for later use.

Marty's Famous Caramels

5 dozen.

1 tablespoon butter
1½ cups white Karo syrup
½ cup butter minus 1 tablespoon
2 cups sugar
2 cups half and half
2 teaspoons vanilla extract
Dash salt

Grease a foil oblong pan with 1 tablespoon butter. In a large kettle, combine Karo syrup and butter. Add sugar and stir until dissolved. Add 1 cup half and half and bring to boil. Remove from heat and add final cup of half and half. Return kettle to heat and bring to a slow boil. When halfway done, approximately 1 hour, add 2 teaspoons vanilla and a dash of salt.

When caramel reaches a firm ball stage, remove from fire and let stand until bubbling stops. Pour into pan. Mixture should be cold before cutting. Can be frozen.

Caramelitas

24 servings.

1 14 ounce package caramels
½ cup evaporated milk
2 cups flour
2 cups oatmeal
1½ cups brown sugar, packed
1 teaspoon baking soda
½ teaspoon salt
1 cup melted butter
1 cup semi-sweet chocolate chips

Melt caramels with milk in double boiler. Cool slightly. Blend flour, oatmeal, brown sugar, baking soda and salt. Add butter. Press half of crumb mixture into greased 9″ x 13″ pan. Bake at 350 degrees for 10 minutes.

Remove from oven and sprinkle with chocolate chips. Spread carefully with caramel mixture. Spread remaining oatmeal mixture on top. Pat well. Bake another 20 minutes or until golden brown. Cool or chill for 1-2 hours. Cut into bars.

Caramel Corn

7 to 10 quarts.

2 cups brown sugar, packed
1 cup butter
½ cup light corn syrup
1 teaspoon salt
1 teaspoon baking soda
1 tablespoon vanilla extract
7½-10 quarts popped popcorn

Place brown sugar, butter, corn syrup and salt in oversized saucepan. Bring to a boil. Reduce heat to boil gently for 5 minutes, stirring constantly. Remove from heat and mix in the baking soda and vanilla. Mixture will become foamy and increase in volume. In large bowl, mix well with popped corn.

Pile on 2 or 3 large cookie sheets (a very large turkey roaster works well) and place in 200 degree oven for 1 hour. Switch position of cookie sheets in the oven half-way through time or stir if in roasting pan.

Microwave Peanut Brittle

8 to 10 servings.

1 cup dry roasted unsalted peanuts
½ cup white corn syrup
1 cup granulated sugar
1 teaspoon butter or margarine
1 teaspoon vanilla extract
¼ teaspoon salt
1 teaspoon baking soda

In 4 cup glass container (measuring cup works well) mix the first 3 ingredients. Microwave mixture on high for 4 minutes then remove and add the next three ingredients. Stir well and microwave mixture on high for 1 minute 30 seconds. Add 1 teaspoon baking soda and gently stir until light and foamy.

Pour mixture onto lightly greased cookie sheet. Bake in preheated 250 degree oven for 5 minutes. Allow to cool (30-60 minutes) and then break into small pieces. Store in an airtight container.

Fudge Peanut Blossoms

3 dozen.

1⅓ cups sweetened condensed milk
2 12 ounce packages peanut butter flavored chips
½ teaspoon orange extract
Chopped nuts
Granulated sugar
1 9 ounce package milk chocolate kisses, unwrapped

Combine milk and chips in double boiler over warm water. Heat until smooth. If desired, blend in orange extract. Pour into buttered 9″ square pan. Cool. Shape into 1″ balls, roll in nuts or granulated sugar. Press unwrapped chocolate kiss into center of each ball. Do not refrigerate.

Chocolate Truffles

50 pieces.

1⅔ cups heavy cream
7 tablespoons unsalted butter
1 pound semi-sweet chocolate, cut or broken into pieces
2 tablespoons Grand Marnier
Cocoa powder

Place cream and butter in saucepan. Let butter melt over medium heat. Then, stirring all the while, turn up the heat and let cream just come to a boil. Remove from heat. Add chocolate to saucepan and stir until it is completely melted. Continue stirring until the mixture thickens and cools somewhat. Stir in Grand Marnier, cover mixture and place in refrigerator. Let the mixture thicken for at least 2 hours, stirring 3-4 times as it cools and hardens.

To form truffles, scoop up portions of the chocolate with a spoon. Dust surface thickly with cocoa. Then with cocoa-dusted palms, roll the chocolate portions between your hands to make balls. Roll the balls in cocoa. Refrigerate again immediately.

Brownies

36 bars.

½ pound butter
4 squares semi-sweet chocolate
1 cup brown sugar
1 cup sugar
4 eggs
1½ cups chopped nuts
2 cups flour
2 teaspoons vanilla extract

Melt butter and chocolate in double boiler. Turn off heat. Add sugars and stir. Add eggs and stir. Combine nuts, flour and vanilla and add to mixture. Mix by hand. Thinly spread mixture in jellyroll pan. Bake in 350 degree oven for 10 minutes.

Cream Cheese Brownies

16 brownies.

2 1 ounce squares unsweetened
   chocolate
½ cup butter
1 cup sugar
2 eggs, beaten
1 teaspoon vanilla extract
¼ cup flour
¼ teaspoon salt
½ cup coarsely chopped nuts
1 3 ounce package cream cheese,
   cut into ½″ cubes
1 6 ounce package semi-sweet
   chocolate pieces

Melt chocolate and butter in heavy saucepan or microwave in glass bowl. Remove from heat and stir in sugar. Add eggs and vanilla. Stir in flour, salt and nuts until blended. Turn batter into buttered 8″ x 8″ pan. Drop in cubes of cream cheese. Bake at 325 degrees for 35-40 minutes. Quickly sprinkle chocolate pieces all over top and return to oven and bake 3 more minutes. Remove and spread chocolate while warm. Cool and cut into squares or bars.

Heavenly Sinful Brownies

2 dozen.

1 cup sugar
½ cup butter
4 eggs, beaten
1 cup flour
½ teaspoon salt
1 16 ounce can chocolate syrup
1 teaspoon vanilla extract
2 cups powdered sugar
½ cup butter
2 tablespoons green creme de menthe
1 cup chocolate chips
6 tablespoons butter

Cream sugar and butter. Add eggs. Add next 4 ingredients in order given. Blend well. Pour into greased 9″ x 13″ pan. Bake in preheated 350 degree oven for 35-40 minutes.

For middle layer, mix powdered sugar with butter and creme de menthe. Spread on cooled cake.

For glaze, melt chocolate chips with butter. Let cool until it will spread evenly over cake and middle layer. Chill and cut into squares.

Chocolate Mocha Bran Brownies

16 bars.

3 tablespoons cocoa powder
1 tablespoon instant coffee
1 tablespoon water
2 very ripe bananas
2 cups sugar
6 egg whites
1 teaspoon vanilla extract
1 cup oat bran cereal
¼ teaspoon salt (optional)
1 cup chopped nuts or raisins

Combine the cocoa, coffee, water and bananas and mix in a blender or a large bowl with a hand mixer. Add the sugar, egg whites, vanilla and mix well. Sift together the oatbran cereal and salt, then add to the mixture. Fold in the nuts. Pour into a 9″ baking pan coated with oil and flour or just a no-stick cooking spray.

Bake in 350 degree oven for 45 minutes. Cut into individual squares, cool and serve.

Scotch Shortbread

3 to 4 dozen.

1 cup butter
½ cup plus 2 tablespoons sugar
1 egg yolk
3 cups sifted flour

Cream butter until soft. Gradually add sugar and continue beating until light and fluffy. Add egg yolk. Add flour in three additions. Divide mixture in half and on lightly floured board, roll out each half to ½″ thickness. Place in pans and score dough in squares. Pierce each square with a fork.

Bake for 25 minutes in 325 degree oven. Cool and separate into pieces.

Forgotten Cookies

3 dozen.

2 egg whites at room temperature
1 cup super fine sugar
1 teaspoon peppermint flavoring
1½ cups chocolate chips

Before beginning preparation, preheat oven to 350 degrees. Whip egg whites to heavy consistency. Add sugar slowly and beat until peaks form. Fold in flavoring and chips. Drop by teaspoonfuls onto ungreased cookie sheets. Put sheets in oven and turn off immediately. Without opening oven door, leave in for at least 5 hours or overnight.

No Sugar Orange-Oatmeal Cookies

2 dozen.

½ cup butter, room temperature
1 egg
6 ounces frozen unsweetened orange juice concentrate, thawed
1 cup flour
¼ teaspoon salt
1 teaspoon baking powder
1 cup oats
½ cup walnuts
½ cup golden raisins

Cream together butter and egg until well mixed. Gradually beat in juice concentrate. Combine flour, salt, baking powder, oats, walnuts and raisins in large bowl. Stir well. Mix dry ingredients and creamed mixture together. Drop by large teaspoons 2″ apart onto greased baking sheet. Bake in 350 degree oven for 15-17 minutes.

§ *Calories: 73 Fat: 3.9gm Cholesterol: 12mg Sodium: 53mg*

Best Sugar Cookies

4 dozen.

1 cup butter or margarine
1 cup powdered sugar
1 cup granulated sugar
2 eggs
1 cup oil
2 teaspoons vanilla extract
1 teaspoon baking soda
1 teaspoon cream of tartar
½ teaspoon salt
5 cups flour

Cream butter with powdered sugar and 1 cup granulated sugar. Beat in eggs until smooth. Slowly stir in oil, vanilla, baking soda, cream of tartar, salt and flour. Chill for easy handling. Shape into walnut-size balls. Dip in granulated sugar. Place on baking sheet and press down. Bake at 350 degrees for 10-12 minutes.

Double Chocolate Chip Cookies

3 dozen.

1¾ cups flour
¼ teaspoon baking soda
½ cup butter
½ cup Crisco or butter-flavored Crisco
1 teaspoon vanilla extract
1 cup sugar
½ cup dark brown sugar, firmly packed
1 egg
⅓ cup unsweetened cocoa
2 tablespoons milk
1 cup semi-sweet chocolate chips

Combine flour and baking soda and set aside. Cream butter and Crisco by hand or electric mixer. Add vanilla and sugars and beat until fluffy. Beat in the egg. Slowly beat in cocoa and then add milk. Stir in flour mixture. Fold in chocolate chips. Drop dough onto cookie sheet by rounded teaspoons and bake at 350 degrees for 12-13 minutes.

Remove from oven and allow to cool slightly before removing from cookie sheet.

Chocolate Chip Pudding Cookies

2 dozen.

2¼ cups flour
1 teaspoon baking soda
1 cup margarine, softened
¼ cup sugar
¾ cup light brown sugar
1 4 ounce package vanilla instant pudding mix
1 teaspoon vanilla extract
1 teaspoon black walnut extract
2 eggs
1 6 ounce package chocolate chips
1 cup chopped nuts (optional)

Mix flour with baking soda. Combine margarine, sugars, pudding mix and extract in a large mixing bowl. Beat until smooth and creamy. Beat in eggs. Gradually add flour mixture, then stir in chocolate chips and nuts. Batter will be stiff. Drop by teaspoonfuls on greased cookie sheets and bake in 375 degree oven for 8-10 minutes.

Easy Cookies

4 dozen.

2 cups sugar
½ cup milk
½ cup butter
¼ cup cocoa
3 cups rolled oats
¼ cup crunchy peanut butter
1 teaspoon vanilla extract

Combine sugar, milk, butter and cocoa together in a saucepan and boil for 2 minutes. In a mixing bowl, combine rolled oats, peanut butter and vanilla. Pour milk mixture over oats and blend thoroughly. Drop the batter from a teaspoon on wax paper to cool.

Lemon-Pecan Cookies

5½ dozen.

1½ cups butter or margarine
1 cup powdered sugar
2½ cups flour
½ cup ground pecans
½ teaspoon salt
1 teaspoon lemon juice
4 tablespoons finely ground lemon rind

Cream butter and powdered sugar. Add next 5 ingredients and blend well. After mixing ingredients, form into ½″ rolls. Wrap in wax paper and chill. Cut rolls into slices ¼″ thick. Place on baking sheets. Bake at 325 degrees for 20 minutes just until golden brown. Freezes beautifully.

Peanut Butter Cookies

4 dozen.

½ cup butter or margarine
½ cup peanut butter
½ cup granulated sugar
½ cup brown sugar
1 egg
½ teaspoon vanilla extract
¼ cup sifted all-purpose flour
¾ teaspoon soda
¼ teaspoon salt

Thoroughly cream butter, peanut butter, sugars, egg and vanilla. Sift together dry ingredients; blend into creamed mixture. Shape into 1″ balls. Place 2″ apart on ungreased cookie sheet. Press with fork tines. Bake in 375 degree oven for 10-12 minutes. Cool slightly; remove from pan.

Child's Play Peanut Butter Cookies

2½ dozen.

2 cups peanut butter
2 cups sugar
2 eggs

Combine all ingredients. Drop on ungreased cookie sheet. Bake in 350 degree oven for 10 minutes.

Holiday Cut Outs

5 dozen.

1 cup butter or margarine
1 cup sugar
1 egg
2 teaspoons vanilla extract
2⅔ cups flour
Egg whites
Food coloring

Cream butter and gradually add sugar, creaming well. Blend in egg and vanilla. Gradually add flour. Mix well. Form dough into a ball, wrap in waxed paper and put in refrigerator for at least 2 hours. Roll dough out on a floured surface. Cut into shapes with cookie cutters. Place on ungreased cookie sheet.

Beat one egg white for each different color. Add food coloring to egg white. Brush on color. Bake for 7-10 minutes in 375 degree oven.

Apricot Horns

11 dozen.

1 pound butter or margarine
1 pound creamed cottage cheese
4 cups sifted flour (approximately)
1 pound dried apricots
2 cups sugar
1½ cups ground almonds
1¼ cups sugar
2 egg whites, slightly beaten
Powdered sugar

Blend butter, cottage cheese and flour together with hands to form dough. Add more flour if cheese is watery. Shape into 1″ balls and refrigerate overnight. (Dough can be kept under refrigeration for one month).

To make filling, cook apricots in water until tender; drain and puree. Combine with sugar while still hot. Cool.

Mix nuts with 1¼ cups sugar. Roll each dough ball into a 3″ round (make only 10 horns at a time so remainder of dough will stay cold). Place a teaspoon of apricot filling in center. Roll up in the shape of a horn. Dip into egg white and then roll in nut mixture. Place on a greased baking sheet. Bake in 375 degree oven for 12 minutes or until lightly browned. Sprinkle with powdered sugar.

Chocolate Chip Cheese Squares

24 squares.

2 packages refrigerated chocolate chip cookie dough
2 8 ounce packages cream cheese
1 egg
1 teaspoon vanilla extract
⅓ cup sugar

Slice 1 package of cookie dough and layer on bottom of a 9″ x 13″ pan. Mix cream cheese, egg, vanilla and sugar. Spread over cookie dough. Slice remaining package of cookie dough and layer on top. Bake in 350 degree oven for 35 minutes. Cool and slice into squares.

Neiman Marcus Squares

4 dozen bars.

½ cup melted margarine
1 18.25 ounce package yellow cake mix
3 eggs
1 8 ounce package cream cheese, softened
16 ounces powdered sugar
½ cup flaked coconut
½ cup chopped walnuts or pecans

Combine margarine, cake mix and 1 egg. Stir together until dry ingredients are moistened. Pat mixture into bottom of well greased 15″ x 10″ jellyroll pan.

Beat remaining 2 eggs lightly, then beat in cream cheese and powdered sugar. Stir in coconut and nuts. Pour over mixture in jellyroll pan, spreading evenly. Bake at 325 degrees 45-50 minutes or until golden brown. Cool pan on wire rack to room temperature, cut into bars to serve.

Oatmeal Crispies

3 dozen.

1 cup margarine, softened
1 cup brown sugar
1 cup sugar
2 eggs, beaten
1 teaspoon vanilla extract
1½ cups flour
1 teaspoon salt
1 teaspoon baking soda
3 cups oatmeal
½ cup chopped walnuts
¼ cup raisins (optional)

Thoroughly cream margarine and sugars. Add eggs and vanilla and beat well.

Sift flour, salt and baking soda and add to creamed mixture. Stir in oatmeal, nuts and raisins. Shape into rolls and wrap in waxed paper and chill.

Cut rolls into ¼″ thick slices. Bake on ungreased cookie sheet in 350 degree oven for 10 minutes.

Peanut Brittle Crunchies

4 dozen.

1¾ cups all-purpose flour
1 cup (2 sticks) butter or margarine, room temperature
½ cup sugar
½ cup light brown sugar
1 teaspoon vanilla extract
1 egg yolk
1 8 ounce package semi-sweet chocolate pieces
⅔ cup salted peanuts, finely chopped

Preheat oven to 275 degrees. Grease a 15½″ x 10½″ jellyroll pan.

Into large bowl, add first 6 ingredients. With mixer at low speed, beat until well blended, scraping with rubber spatula. Spread dough evenly in pan. Bake for 1 hour 10 minutes or until golden. About 10 minutes before cookies are done, in heavy 1 quart saucepan over low heat, melt chocolate pieces, stirring frequently. Remove saucepan from heat. Remove cookies from oven. Pour melted chocolate over baked layer in pan. With metal spatula, quickly and evenly spread chocolate over baked layer. Sprinkle with peanuts. Carefully press peanuts into chocolate.

Immediately cut lengthwise into 4 strips. Then cut each strip crosswise into 12 pieces. Cool in pan on wire rack until chocolate is firm. Store bars in airtight container.

Aunt Bea's French Lace Crisps

4 dozen.

⅔ cup brown sugar, packed
½ cup light corn syrup
½ cup shortening
1 cup flour
1 cup finely chopped nuts

Boil brown sugar, syrup and shortening, stirring constantly. Remove from heat. Stir in flour and nuts. Keep batter warm over hot water. Drop by teaspoonfuls about 3″ apart onto lightly greased cookie sheet. Bake in 375 degree oven until set (about 5 minutes). Let stand 3-5 minutes. Remove from cookie sheet.

Cheesy Lemon Bars

36 bars.

1 package lemon cake mix
½ cup butter or margarine, melted
1 egg
1 package lemon frosting mix
1 8 ounce package cream cheese, softened
2 eggs

Preheat oven to 350 degrees. Grease bottom only of a 9″ x 13″ pan. Combine cake mix, butter and 1 egg. Stir until moist. Pat into pan. Blend frosting mix and softened cream cheese. Reserve ½ cup of this mixture for frosting the bars when done. Add 2 eggs to the remaining frosting mixture. Beat 3-5 minutes at high speed. Spread over cake mixture in pan and bake at 350 degrees for 30- 40 minutes. Cool, frost and cut into bars.

Lemon-Lime Bars

4 dozen.

2 cups flour
½ cup powdered sugar
1 cup butter
4 eggs
2 cups granulated sugar
Dash of salt
⅓ cup fresh lemon or lime juice
Powdered sugar

In a bowl, combine flour and ½ cup powdered sugar. Cut in butter. Press mixture into 9″ x 13″ baking pan. Bake in 350 degree oven for 20-25 minutes or until golden.

Meanwhile, beat eggs at high speed with electric mixer until light and pale yellow. Gradually add sugar and salt, then juice, continuing to beat at high speed. Pour over hot crust and return to oven. Bake an additional 20-25 minutes until golden. After removing from oven, sprinkle entire top with powdered sugar at once. Cool and cut into bars.

Oatmeal Bars

24 bars.

1 cup softened margarine
1 cup brown sugar
2 cups oatmeal
2 cups sifted flour
½ teaspoon salt
½ teaspoon baking soda
1 teaspoon vanilla extract
Apricot or any other flavor jam

Cream margarine and sugar. Add dry ingredients and vanilla. Pat half of the dough into 9″ x 13″ pan and then spread with jam. Top with remaining half of dough and pat firmly. Bake in 350 degree oven for approximately 25 minutes. Cool and cut into bars.

London Bars

2 dozen bars.

½ cup butter
½ cup brown sugar
1 cup flour

Cream butter, add sugar and flour. Mix ingredients thoroughly and spread in square 9″ x 9″ baking pan. Bake in preheated 375 degree oven for 10 minutes.

Topping:
2 eggs
1 cup brown sugar
3 tablespoons flour
½ teaspoon salt
1 cup chopped nuts
1½ cups shredded coconut
1 teaspoon vanilla extract

Topping:
Beat eggs until light. Add sugar, flour, salt and mix well. Add nuts, coconut, vanilla. Mix thoroughly. Spread over first baked mixture and bake at 375 degrees for 20-30 minutes longer. Cut in squares or strips.

Yummy Bars

24 bars.

1 18.25 ounce box yellow butter cake mix (do not use pudding mix)
1 egg, beaten
½ cup butter, melted
1 8 ounce package cream cheese
3 eggs
¾ pound powdered sugar
1 teaspoon vanilla extract

To cake mix add egg and melted butter to make dough. Press into a 9″ x 13″ pan. Do not bake. Whip the cream cheese and add the eggs, powdered sugar and vanilla. Pour over dough. Bake in 325 degree oven for 1 hour. Top should be lightly brown. Cut into 1½″ squares before completely cooled.

Persimmon Lemon Bars

36 bars.

1   cup persimmon pulp
1½   teaspoons lemon juice
1   teaspoon baking soda
1   egg
⅔   cup sugar
½   cup salad oil
8   ounces pitted dates, chopped fine
1¾   cups unsifted flour
1   teaspoon salt
1   teaspoon cinnamon
¼   teaspoon cloves
1   cup chopped nuts

Lemon Glaze:
1   cup powdered sugar
2   tablespoons lemon juice

Mix pulp with the lemon juice and soda, set aside. In large bowl, beat egg, stir in sugar, oil and dates. Combine flour with other dry ingredients except nuts and add to date mixture alternately with the pulp. Blend well and stir in nuts. Spread in greased and floured 10″ x 15″ jellyroll pan. Bake in 350 degree oven for 25 minutes or until lightly browned. Cool 5 minutes and then coat with Lemon Glaze. Cut into bars.

Lemon Glaze:
Blend 1 cup powdered sugar with 2 tablespoons lemon juice until smooth and spread on bars.

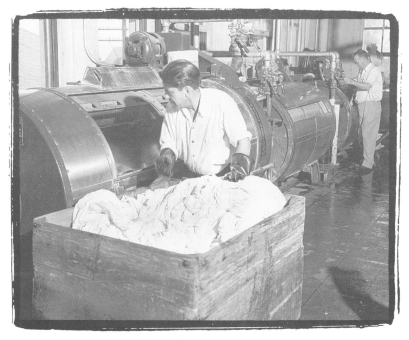

Laundry, 1947

restaurant chef's favorites

Spiced Beef Relish

Take two pounds of raw, tender beef steak, chop it very fine, put into it salt, pepper

and a little sage, two tablespoonfuls of melted butter; add two finely rolled crackers, also

two well-beaten eggs. Make it up into the shape of a roll and bake it; baste

with butter and water before baking. Cut in slices when cold.

The White House Cookbook ©1887

❧

Chilled Watermelon Soup

6 servings.

½ medium red seedless watermelon,
pureed and strained
½ small yellow watermelon, seeded,
cut into ¼″ cubes
(If unable to find yellow watermelon,
substitute 1 cantaloupe)
8 green onions, finely diced
6 sprigs mint leaves, finely diced
3 limes, juice only
Tabasco sauce to taste

Mix all of the ingredients and chill.

Chez Melange, Redondo Beach.

Almost Flourless Chocolate Cake

14 servings.

2 pounds bittersweet chocolate,
melted
10 ounces unsalted butter,
room temperature
8 eggs, separated
Pinch salt
2 tablespoons sugar
2 tablespoons flour

Whisk chocolate and butter until blended. Whip egg yolks until pale yellow, about 5 minutes. Beat whites with pinch of salt. Then add 2 tablespoons of sugar. Beat for 5 seconds. Fold chocolate and egg yolks together, then fold egg whites into chocolate.

Butter sides and bottom of a 10″ pan, cover bottom with paper. Bake in 425 degree oven for 15 minutes. Cake will be soft. Cool completely before removing from pan.

Chez Melange, Redondo Beach.

Papaya Crab Quesadilla with Farmer's Pot Cheese & Roasted Tomato Salsa

4 servings.

1 cup thinly sliced papaya
4 ounces farmer's pot cheese, grated
4 ounces dungeness crab, leg meat
3 tablespoons snipped cilantro
3 green onions, chopped
4 flour tortillas

Roasted Tomato Salsa:
1 cup chicken broth
1 dried Ancho chile, seeded
2 dried Pasilla chiles, seeded
1 dried New Mexican chile, seeded
3 small tomatoes
4 tomatillos
¼ cup cilantro
3 whole cloves garlic
¼ onion, chopped
Salt and pepper

Combine first 5 ingredients. Divide filling equally among the four tortillas. Fold the filled tortillas in half; bake at 350 degrees for 8-10 minutes or until lightly browned. Slice into 4 equal parts per serving. Serve with Roasted Tomato Salsa.

Roasted Tomato Salsa:
Heat chicken stock in small pan; add chiles and simmer until chiles soften, about 5 minutes. Set aside.

Place the tomatoes and tomatillos on a baking sheet and roast in a 425 degree oven until dark brown blisters form on them, about 20 minutes. Combine remaining ingredients with the dry chiles and chicken broth mixture and chop in food processor to reach desired consistency. Add salt and pepper to taste. Add more chicken stock if the salsa is too thick.

Chez Melange, Redondo Beach.

244

Lamb, Orzo &
Roasted Vegetable Salad

8 to 10 servings.

2 medium eggplants,
cut into ½″ pieces
2 red bell peppers, cut into ½″ pieces
2 yellow bell peppers,
cut into ½″ pieces
1 cup olive oil
1 pound orzo
12 ounces feta cheese, crumbled
1 bunch green onions, minced
½ cup chopped fresh mint leaves
⅓ cup pine nuts, lightly toasted
1 cup Kalamata olives, pitted
4 cups lamb, grilled,
cut into chunks or strips
½ cup fresh lemon juice
⅔ cup olive oil
Salt and pepper
Fresh thyme

Place eggplant and bell peppers in mixing bowl. Mix with garlic and olive oil. Roast vegetables on sheet pan in 375 degree oven for 45 minutes or until soft and lightly blistered.

Cook orzo in 3 times the water, strain and run cold water over it to remove the starch.

In a large mixing bowl, place crumbled feta cheese, green onion, mint leaves, pine nuts, Kalamata olives and cooked lamb. Add roasted vegetables and toss with lemon/olive oil vinaigrette. Season to taste with salt and pepper and garnish with fresh thyme.

The Kitchen for Exploring Food, Pasadena.

Baked Salmon with Tequila, Tomato & Basil Vinaigrette

4 servings.

1 ounce tequila
1 ounce white vinegar
1 ounce shallots, julienne fine
1 garlic clove, julienne fine
1 ounce extra virgin olive oil
1 cup tomatoes, diced medium, seeded and cored
2 tablespoons chopped basil
1 poblano pepper, seeded, cored and chopped small
2 tablespoons finely chopped yellow pepper
Juice of 1 lemon
Salt and pepper to taste

Baked Salmon:
24 ounces fresh salmon, skinned and pinned out.
Basil, to taste
Mint, to taste
Dill, to taste
Garlic, fresh chopped, to taste
White pepper, to taste
Salt, to taste
Extra virgin olive oil, to taste

Mix all ingredients together and set aside.

Baked Salmon:
Cut salmon in 4 equal parts and coat lightly with herbs, garlic, pepper, salt and olive oil. Place on cookie sheet and refrigerate for approximately 1 hour.

Set oven to 400 degrees. Place salmon in oven and cook for 5 minutes or until desired doneness is reached. Arrange salmon on plates, pour vinaigrette on salmon. Serve immediately with Jicama Salad, if desired.

Parkway Grill, Pasadena. Executive Chef, Hugo Molina.

Jicama Salad

4 servings.

**1 small jicama,
peeled and julienne fine
4 ounces watercress, stems removed
Juice of 2 lemons
Salt, to taste
Pepper, to taste**

Mix jicama with the watercress. Add lemon juice, salt and pepper. Toss salad and refrigerate until flavors are blended, approximately 1 hour.

Parkway Grill, Pasadena. Executive Chef, Hugo Molina.

Chicken Piccata

6 servings.

**3 chicken breasts, split in 2,
skinned and boned
2 eggs, beaten
2 tablespoons olive oil
Juice from 1 lemon
3-4 fresh basil leaves
½ cup whipping cream
½ cup unsalted butter**

With mallet, pound chicken breast until ¼″ thick. Dip chicken in beaten eggs. In skillet, heat olive oil and cook chicken on both sides until done. Set aside and keep warm. In saucepan, squeeze juice from lemon, add basil and cream. Heat until thickened; reduce temperature and slowly add butter while stirring constantly. Transfer sauce to top of double boiler and beat until creamy. Strain sauce and serve over chicken breasts.

*The Athenaeum, Cal Tech, Pasadena.
Executive Chef, Jean-Pierre Couly.*

Chicken Fajitas

14 servings.

2 pounds chicken, cut into thin strips
2 cups broccoli, cut into 1" pieces
2 cups sliced onions
2 cups sliced green peppers
4 tablespoons soy sauce
4 tablespoons dry sherry
2 teaspoons cornstarch
1 teaspoon sugar
1 cup bean sprouts
Lettuce
7 pita breads, cut in half

Saute chicken strips in hot oil along with broccoli, onions and green peppers. When the chicken is done, add soy sauce, sherry, cornstarch and sugar and mix together well.

Wash and drain bean sprouts and thinly slice some lettuce. Put a small amount of each in a pita bread and then spoon in the chicken fajitas mixture.

The Fox's Restaurant, Altadena.

Poblano Chile Relleno with Roasted Tomato Sauce

4 servings.

4 Poblano or Pasilla peppers
4 ounces lean pork meat, diced small
2 tablespoons chopped fresh garlic
2 ounces red onion, diced small
⅛ cup corn oil
2 ounces zucchini, diced small
½ teaspoon kosher salt
½ teaspoon white pepper
2 ounces corn kernels, cooked
8 ounces asadero or Monterey Jack cheese
4 tablespoons chopped cilantro
2 tablespoons chopped basil

Chile Relleno:

Roast peppers over direct flame until darkened, then make a small cut (lengthwise) in center of pepper, leaving stems intact. Put them under running water to remove skin and seeds.

Saute pork, garlic and onions in corn oil for about 2 minutes. Add zucchini and cook for 2 more minutes. Add salt and pepper.

Remove from heat and strain, discard any liquid. Refrigerate. When pork mixture is completely chilled, mix in corn kernels, asadero cheese, cilantro and basil. Fill pepper with mixture fairly tight.

Roasted Tomato Sauce:
12 ounces fresh whole tomatoes, roasted
4 ounces tomatillo, roasted
2 Guajillo peppers, no stems or seeds
¼ cup orange juice
½ white onion, minced
3 garlic cloves, minced
1½ ounces lard or corn oil
1½ cups chicken broth

Set oven at 400 degrees. Place pepper into 2″ deep pan with 4 ounces water so that peppers won't burn or stick to the pan. Put in oven and cook for about 5 minutes or until totally hot.

Pour roasted tomato sauce on bottom of plates. Place 1 chile relleno on center of plate. Decorate plate around relleno with cheese, green onions, and corn kernels. Serve immediately.

Roasted Tomato Sauce:
Place tomatoes, tomatillos, Guajillo peppers and orange juice in blender. Blend coarsely. Meanwhile saute onions and garlic until dark brown in lard or corn oil. Add tomato mixture. Cook for about 2 minutes, then add chicken broth and cook for about 10 minutes at medium heat or until liquid is reduced to about half.

Crocodile Cantina, Glendale. Executive Chef, Hugo Molina.

Sweet & Pungent Shrimp

6 servings.

2 pounds (size 36/40) raw shrimp
1 egg white
2 cups cornstarch
1 teaspoon salt
3-4 cups vegetable oil (for frying)

Sweet and Pungent Sauce:
4½ tablespoons sugar
4½ tablespoons catsup
4 tablespoons vinegar
½ teaspoon salt
1 tablespoon sherry
½ teaspoon cornstarch
1 teaspoon oil to coat pan
2 large garlic cloves, minced
¾ teaspoon minced fresh ginger
1 tablespoon chopped green onion
1 teaspoon crushed red pepper
1 teaspoon zest of lemon
1 teaspoon zest of orange

Peel and devein shrimp. Slice in half lengthwise. Rinse well and blot with towel to remove excess water. Add egg white and mix well. Mix 3 tablespoons cornstarch and salt together and add to shrimp; mix well. Add 1½ tablespoons vegetable oil and mix well again. Place shrimp in bowl and refrigerate for at least 2 hours.

Remove shrimp from refrigerator and dust with remaining cornstarch. Shrimp should be dry to the touch. Heat oil in wok until very hot (350-375 degrees). Fry shrimp, taking care to separate shrimp with long handled wooden spoon or chop sticks to avoid sticking together. It may be necessary to fry shrimp in several batches so oil does not cool down. Fry for about 1½-2 minutes until crisp. Remove shrimp from oil with long handled strainer and drain well.

Prepare Sweet and Pungent Sauce and add to shrimp, stirring quickly to coat shrimp. Immediately turn out onto platter and sprinkle with finely chopped green onion.

Sweet and Pungent Sauce:
Mix sugar, catsup, vinegar and salt; set aside. Mix sherry and cornstarch; set aside. Heat 1 teaspoon oil in wok. Add garlic, ginger, onion, red pepper and zests of lemon and orange. Cook about 30 seconds. Stir in sugar/catsup mixture. Immediately add sherry/cornstarch mixture and cook briefly to thicken.

Panda Inn, Pasadena.

Paella

8 to 12 servings.

3 cups rice, uncooked
16 chicken legs and/or
2nd joints/breasts
½ pound Italian sausage (mild or hot)
½ pound pork chorizo
1 large onion, thinly sliced
2 bay leaves
1 clove garlic, chopped finely
⅛ teaspoon saffron
1 cup white wine
½ gallon chicken stock,
cooked and kept hot
1 pound clams or shrimp, may vary
amount depending upon personal taste
Salt and pepper to taste
¼ pound ham cut in strips
(for garnish)
12-15 black olives, sliced
(for garnish)

Soak rice overnight, drain and set aside.

Saute chicken with sausage, chorizo and onion for 5 minutes. Add rice, bay leaves, garlic, saffron, wine and chicken stock. Stir until blended. Bake in 375 degree oven for 30 minutes. Five minutes before removing from oven add fresh seafood, any kind you select. Make sure the seafood is cut in bite-size pieces. Salt and pepper dish to taste. Garnish with ham and black olives.

The Chronicle, Pasadena.

Russian Style Smoked Salmon

2 servings as appetizer; 1 serving as main course.

¼ cup salad oil
½ bunch fresh parsley leaves
¼ cup all-purpose flour
¼ large onion, sliced thin
1 medium potato,
peeled and thinly sliced
1 ounce sour cream
3½-4 ounces smoked salmon,
sliced thin
½ lemon or 2 lemon wedges
½ ounce caviar (optional)

Heat the oil on top of stove to about 325-350 degrees. Working quickly, dust parsley leaves in flour, and fry. Remove, and put onion slices in flour, quickly fry, remove from heat. Do the same procedure for the potato slices, fry until crispy.

To serve, place fried potatoes in the middle of the plate, topped with sour cream. Put half of the fried onion, then fried parsley, with another layer of potatoes and sour cream. Cover the remaining layer with the smoked salmon. Garnish with lemon wedges and caviar if desired.

The Chronicle, Pasadena.

Mackey's Garlic Mashed Potatoes

20 servings.

Mashed Potatoes:
5 pounds russet potatoes
6 ounces butter
6 ounces milk
Salt and pepper to taste

Garlic Butter:
7 ounces garlic, peeled
1¼ pound plus 1 tablespoon butter,
softened

Mashed Potatoes:
Peel, dice and boil potatoes. Drain and mash. Mix well with remaining ingredients. Add garlic butter to mashed potatoes, about 1-2 tablespoons per serving.

Garlic Butter:
Saute peeled garlic in one ounce butter. Roast in 350 degree oven until golden brown (about 20-30 minutes). Cool and whip with softened butter.

Mackey's Restaurant, Pasadena.

Broiled Jumbo Scallops with Red Bell Pepper Sauce & Linguini with Pine Nuts

2 servings.

2 red bell peppers
3 tablespoons olive oil
1 small onion, peeled and cut rough
1 tablespoon chopped garlic
2 tablespoons chopped shallots
1 cup port wine
2 cups chicken stock or broth
¼ cup tomato sauce
Salt and pepper
10 jumbo scallops or approximately
12 ounces bay scallops
4 ounces linguini
¼ cup roasted pine nuts
2 blue corn tortillas (julienne)

Rough chop peppers and remove seeds. Heat olive oil and saute peppers, onion, garlic and shallots until soft. Add port wine and reduce to half. Add chicken stock and tomato sauce. Let cook on medium boil for 20 minutes. Place contents in blender or food processor and puree, add salt and pepper to taste and hold warm.

If broiling or barbecuing, lightly oil and season scallops. If pan sauteing scallops, they should be dusted with flour lightly and cooked with olive oil in very hot pan.

Cook linguini and toss with red bell pepper sauce and pine nuts. Place linguini on plate and place scallops around plate close to border leaving the middle open for more sauce and julienne strips of blue corn tortillas for garnish.

Restaurant Lozano, Sierra Madre.

Mackey's Mint Sauce

2 cups.

1 cup white vinegar
½ cup sugar
1 tablespoon cornstarch
1 cup chopped fresh mint
2 cloves garlic, chopped
1 teaspoon chopped rosemary

Boil vinegar and sugar. Add cornstarch mixed with enough water to make a paste. Return to boil and pour over mint leaves, garlic and rosemary. Serve with lamb or fish.

Mackey's Restaurant, Pasadena.

Tortilla Soup

10 servings

3 tablespoons olive oil
1 whole white or yellow onion, diced
2 tablespoons minced garlic
3 whole red bell peppers, diced and seeded
1 tablespoon whole cumin
1 quart chicken stock
1 tablespoon chicken base
1 quart fresh tomato puree (12-15 blanched peeled tomatoes)
1 quart canned tomato puree
1 bunch fresh cilantro, chopped
4 bay leaves
2 tablespoons tabasco sauce
1 tablespoon Mexican oregano
1 tablespoon fresh thyme

In large heavy skillet, heat olive oil and saute the onion, garlic, red peppers and cumin until tender, but not brown.

In a large soup pot, combine the chicken stock, chicken base, tomato puree, fresh cilantro, bay leaves, tabasco sauce, oregano, pepper, thyme, rosemary, chipotle chile, sugar and salt. Heat to a boil and lower to simmer. Add the sauteed contents and continue to simmer for about 1 hour 30 minutes.

At this point, one of two things may be done. If a thick soup is desired, remove the rosemary branch and bay leaves and puree in a blender. If a thinner soup is desired, strain through a cheesecloth.

1 tablespoon coarsely ground black pepper
1 6"-8" branch of fresh rosemary
1 tablespoon finely minced chipotle chile (salsa jalapeno may be substituted)
2 tablespoons sugar
1 teaspoon salt
4 corn tortillas
1 bunch cilantro
1 large onion, diced
4 boneless, skinless breasts of chicken
4 whole pasilla or poblano chiles
2 whole avocados
Juice of 1 lemon
4 ounces feta cheese (aged dry jack, or cheddar may be used)

While the soup is simmering prepare the garnishes. Slice corn tortillas into thin julienne strips and deep fry until crisp. Drain. Wash, drain and pick over cilantro and coarse chop. Dice one large onion. Broil or grill chicken breasts until golden brown and cut into julienne strips. Roast chiles directly on top of stove burners until skins crackle and are black. Scrape off skins and remove stems and seeds, and cut into julienne strips. Dice 2 ripe avocados and set aside in a bowl of cold water (just enough to cover) and juice of one lemon. Grate, crumble or shave cheese of your choice.

When soup is ready to serve, add to empty soup bowls a small amount of each garnish except cheese. Ladle soup over all, and top with cheese.

Sonora Cafe, Los Angeles.

Green Street Mustard Vinaigrette

2 cups.

1 cup corn oil
¾ cup vinegar
1 teaspoon tabasco
2 tablespoons Dijon mustard
5 tablespoons HMR mustard
2 teaspoons Italian dressing
Dash salt

Mix all ingredients together well.

Green Street Restaurant, Pasadena.

Green Street Restaurant Meatloaf

12 servings.

1 large onion
1 clove garlic
6½ ounces fresh spinach
4 ounces bread crumbs
2½ pounds ground beef
1 ounce parmesan cheese
2 tablespoons salt
1 tablespoon dried parsley
2 eggs, lightly beaten
Fresh ground pepper to taste
4 ounces Swiss cheese
⅓ pound grated jack cheese
Melted butter

Preheat oven to 350 degrees. Finely chop onion, garlic and spinach in food processor. Generously butter one 12″ x 4″ x 2½″ baking pan. Sprinkle with bread crumbs to coat entire bread pan. In a large bowl, mix well all ingredients except jack cheese, Swiss cheese and melted butter.

Divide meat mixture into three equal portions. Pat one-third of meat mixture into bottom of pan (meat must touch sides of pan). Place Swiss cheese on top of meat. Add second third of meat mixture on top of Swiss cheese, making sure meat touches sides of pan. Place jack cheese on top of second layer of meat. Add final portion of meat mixture on top of jack cheese. Push edges of meat down, so the top is somewhat rounded. Lightly sprinkle with butter on top. Bake for about 1 hour.

Green Street Restaurant, Pasadena.

Sukiyaki

6 servings.

Small piece of suet
(fat from top sirloin)
1½ pounds top sirloin,
sliced bacon thin
⅔ cup celery slices
2 bunches green onions, cut 2″ long
⅔ cup sliced fresh mushrooms
½ No. 2 can bamboo shoots, sliced
½ pound fresh bean sprouts
1½ pounds dry onions, sliced
½ bean curd cake (tofu) sliced
1 cup yam noodles

Sukiyaki Cooking Sauce:
2 ounces Japanese wine (sake)
2 teaspoons sugar
½ cup Japanese soy sauce
½ cup consomme or beef stock

Preheat pan or 12″ skillet, rub bottom with suet, and add vegetables, keeping them in separate groups. Add the meat and the cooking sauce. Turn vegetables and meat over once during cooking. Serve while vegetables are still crisp—with hot steamed rice.

Sukiyaki Cooking Sauce:
Heat and blend until sugar dissolves.

Miyako Restaurant, Pasadena.

257

Chicken Appetizers
& Teriyaki Sauce (Yaki-Tori)

12 servings.

1 2½ pound frying chicken
Flour

Teriyaki Sauce:
1 cup Japanese soy sauce
½ cup sugar
2 teaspoons Japanese wine (sake)
1 tablespoon grated ginger
1 teaspoon cornstarch

Bone chicken completely and cut into small bite-sized pieces-about 35 pieces. Flour chicken pieces thoroughly and deep fry at 350 degrees until done.

Do not dip, but pour teriyaki sauce over fried chicken bits so that a light coating of the sauce will be on each chicken bit. Skewer and serve.

Teriyaki Sauce:
Heat and blend the soy sauce, sugar, sake and ginger. Add cornstarch as the last step, with very little water to thicken the teriyaki sauce.

Miyako Restaurant, Pasadena.

Roasted Garlic Soup

8 servings.

3 heads garlic
1 large onion
1 leek
2 tablespoons olive oil
2 potatoes, peeled and sliced
2 quarts vegetable broth or water
3 or 4 cloves "elephant" garlic
Red bell pepper for garnish
1 cup cream
Salt and pepper

Roast 3 heads of garlic (whole and unpeeled) in a 350 degree oven for 45 minutes. They should be soft and golden brown.

Slice the onion and the white of the leek. Saute in olive oil in a large kettle until soft but not brown. Add the roasted garlic, sliced potatoes and vegetable broth and simmer for 1 hour.

In the meantime, slice the cloves of "elephant" garlic into thin slices to make garlic chips for the garnish. Fry the slices in a little oil for about two minutes until golden brown. Drain on a towel and reserve. Cut the red bell pepper into a pretty julienne and reserve as well.

Just before the soup is done, add the cream, puree and strain the soup. Season with salt and pepper to taste. Pour the soup into bowls and sprinkle with red bell pepper and garlic chips.

La Toque, Los Angeles.

Plantains with Mango Salsa

4 servings.

2 ripe plantains
Sugar (to taste)
Pinch of cinnamon
2 tablespoons olive oil
¼ cup diced red onions
½ cup diced red pepper
1 cup diced mango
1 tablespoon cilantro
Juice from one lime
Sour cream (optional)

Boil plantains for 15 minutes. Remove skin and puree or mash with hands. Add sugar and cinnamon to taste. Make little patties approximately 3″ round and ½″ thick. Refrigerate while waiting for plantains to firm up. In olive oil, saute onions and peppers till soft. Then cool. Add to diced mango, cilantro and juice from lime. To finish plantains, heat a little olive oil in skillet, enough to cover bottom of pan and brown both sides. Place plantains on plate topped with mango salsa and optional sour cream.

Restaurant Lozano, Sierra Madre.

Catavinos Corn & Crab Cakes

5 servings.

10 ounces crab meat
16 ounces corn, pureed
(canned or frozen)
4 tablespoons green onion,
chopped fine
2 tablespoons garlic, chopped fine
¼ cup flour (may be a little more
so mixture looks dry)
1 egg or 2 yolks
1 teaspoon salt
2 egg whites

Cayenne Sherry Mayo:
½ cup mayonnaise
⅛ cup sherry
⅛ cilantro, chopped fine
Cayenne pepper to taste

Mix all of the ingredients except egg whites. Whip whites until stiff, add to mixture. Mold into 10-12 small cakes. Saute in a little oil until lightly browned.

Cayenne Sherry Mayo:
Mix all ingredients together. Serve as sauce for crab cakes.

Catavino, Pasadena.

acknowledgments

The steering committee of "Celebrating the Centennial" wish to thank its members, families and friends who have contributed recipes. It is our sincere hope that no one has been inadvertently overlooked.

Abbott, Julie
Adams, Carolyn
Alexander, Carolyn
Almanza, Graziella
Amagrande, Marie
Amato, Pat
Anderson, Eileen
Anderson, Evelyn
Andrews, Cathy
Anson, Roxana
Ares, Terri
Backer, Jacque
Baer, Sydney
Baker, Sally
Ball, Dorothy
Basore, Doris
Black, Janet
Blond, Marilyn
Bockus, Janet
Bolenbaugh, Judy
Bowdoin, Joan
Boyd, Claudette
Boynes, Adele
Brady, Katherine
Bragg, Martha Ann
Bressler, Melia
Broerman, Elaine
Burns, Anne
Carter, Charmaine
Cathey, Irene

Catron, Kathy
Cobb, Peggy
Conroy, Patti
Corona, Kathleen
Crick, Marty
Crowell, Tina
Dahl, Patricia
Dattola, Dawn
Davidson, Milissa
DeGrassi, Dolores
Dennerline, Barbara
DePaul, Hazel
DePaul, Carole
DePaul, Marie
Deputy, Norma
Devine, Nancy
Dito, Loretta
Duer, Dorothy
Duff, Peggy
Dullo, Frances
Dunne, Jean
DuPree, Brenda
Ehlers, Sandy
Eisenbruch, Rita
Ellis, Helen
Erwin, Diane
Field, Janet
Fisher, Dick
Flores, Cynthia
Forbes, Claudia

Fortune, Virginia
Fox, Carol
Frindt, Clem
Gamb, Priscilla
Gamble, Cathy
Gill, Angela
Gindele, Pearl
Giraino, Marie
Girvetz, Phyllis
Grawet, Brett
Greve, Margaret
Griggs, Barbara
Gunter, Julie
Hamane, Geri
Hartung, Skip
Hawley, Jean Anne
Hayashi, Alice
Hayne, Marion
HMH Dietary Department
Hoge, Claudette
Hoover, Betsy
Hopfinger, Jackie
Hull, Dorothy
Irwin, Diane
James, Anne
Jenkins, Linda
Jick, Bryan
Johnson, Jean
Johnston, Anne
Joseph, Benny

Juett, Dorothy
Kaiser, Ann
Keigel, Fran
Khazoyan, Virginia
Kipnis, Miriam
Knapp, Lois
Krall, Jan
Kritzman, Millie
Krueger, Paula
Kurihara, Leah
Lavender, Merlyn
Leonhard, Wyllis
Levin, Beverly
Levin, Shelly
Lewis, Janet
Logan, Peggy
Longo, Geri
MacInnes, Betty
Mackey, Daphne
MacLaren, Dorothy
Marshall, Dorothy
McCormick, Julie
McCrea, Ruth
McDonald, Grace
Miller, Bobbie
Miller, Dorothy
Miller, Grandma
Morris, Herb
Moulton, Darle
Mugnain, Ruth
Munnecke, Virginia
Nenning, Dee
Newcomer, Elizabeth
Niles, Patricia

Nuremburg, Karen
Packard, Charlotte
Park, Marty
Parker, Clarice
Pasini, Emma
Pavlinek, Mary
Peery, Marjorie
Pelton, R. Allen
Pendleton, Carol
Peschke, Phoebe
Phelps, Evelyn
Powell, Ronald E.
Powell, Alba
Price, Jan Leanne
Price-Lauder, Donna
Pruitt, Judy
Rambeau, Bonita
Reber, Debbie
Reichel-Clark, Cathy
Repetti, Anamaria
Reynolds, Carol
Reynolds, Dani
Reynolds, Jean Carol
Riepe, Suzanne
Rohrlietner, Kathy
Rosier, Jewell
Rounds, Jan
Russell, Peggy
Sadler, Elsie
Sanborn, Gay
Sardisco, Teresa
Satzinger, La Vone
Schetrom, Dolores
Schuele, Kris

Shepro, Eleanor
Simon, Venice
Skelman, Warren
Slater, Alayne
Smelser, Mrs. George
Smith, Ginny
Snowder, Caroline
Snyder, Charlotte
Sorenson, Lois
Sorenson, Patricia
Stalzberg, Sylvia
Stanson, Betty
Stoke, Corrine
Stone, Barbara
Tatro, Jeanne
Thomas, Joan
Thompson, Margaret
Thomson, Evelyn
Thrane, Joanne
Totten, Estelle
Uhlir, Maureen
Verleger, Hester
Weber, Melissa
Weigand, Debbie
Whipple, Jo Anne
White, Nancy
Wood, Millie
Yamamoto, Michiko
Yingling, Peggy
Young, Ginny
Zeilstra, Denise
Zinni, Ellie

index

Seafood Bisque, *68*
Shrimp & Crabmeat Jambalaya, *113*
Shrimp Brew, *109*
Shrimp Chippewa, *112*
Shrimp Stuffed Sole, *112*
Shrimp with Garden Fresh Vegetables & Fruit, *110*
Stir-Fry Seasame Shrimp and Asparagus, *110*
Sweet and Pungent Shrimp, *250*
Tangarine Filet of Sole, *105*

Seafood Bisque, *68*
Seasoned Carrot Bake, *168*
Sherry Mustard Chicken or Turkey, *119*
Shredded Wheat Dessert (Poor Man's Baklava), *217*
Shrimp & Crabmeat Jambalaya, *113*
Shrimp Brew, *109*
Shrimp Chippewa, *112*
Shrimp Stuffed Sole, *112*
Shrimp with Garden Fresh Vegetables & Fruit, *110*
Sir Sydney's Skirt Steak, *139*
Skinny Dip, *24*
Smoked Salmon Log, *21*
Sonoma Chicken Salad, *81*

Soup

Acapulco Vegetarian Soup, *72*
Broccoli Soup, *66*
California Chili, *72*
Chilled Watermelon Soup, *243*
Cold Chili Soup, *65*
Crab Bisque, *71*
Cream Mongole, *74*
Diana's Carrot Soup, *67*
Dieter's Meal-In-One Vegetable Soup, *75*
Ellie's Manhattan Clam Chowder, *76*
Green Soup, *78*

Hearty Harvest Soup, *73*
Hot Tomato Bouillon, *73*
Hungarian Sauerkraut Soup, *78*
Mushroom Soup Supreme, *67*
Portuguese Kale Soup, *77*
Potato, Ham & Cheese Soup, *76*
Potato Leek Soup, *70*
Pumpkin Soup, *66*
Rice-Shrimp Gumbo, *74*
Roasted Garlic Soup, *259*
Seafood Bisque, *68*
Tortilla Soup, *254*
Two Melon Soup, *65*
Winter Vegetable Chowder, *71*
Zucchini Cheese Chowder, *77*
Zucchini Italian Sausage Soup, *69*

Soused Apple Cake, *199*
Spanish Bean Pot, *166*
Spicy Acorn Squash, *177*
Spicy Chicken Vegetable Micro, *128*
Spinach Delight, *176*
Spinach Noodle Ring, *56*
Spinach or Broccoli Casserole, *175*
Spinach/Sprouts & Fruit Salad, *91*
Stir Fry Sesame Shrimp & Asparagus, *110*
Streusel Topping Cupcakes, *207*
Stuffed Shells in Sauce, *184*
Stuffed Sweet Potatoes, *174*
Sukiyaki, *257*
Sumi Salad, *79*
Summer Squash Casserole, *176*
Sunshine Carrots, *169*
Sweet & Pungent Shrimp, *250*
Sweet & Sour Pork, *147*
Swiss Cheese Dip, *23*